COPING WITH
Endometriosis

COPING WITH
Endometriosis

Sound, Compassionate Advice for Alleviating
the Physical and Emotional Symptoms of
This Frequently Misunderstood Illness

ROBERT H. PHILLIPS, PH.D., and
GLENDA MOTTA, R.N., M.P.H.

Avery
A MEMBER OF
PENGUIN PUTNAM INC.
NEW YORK

Most Avery books are available at special quantity discounts for bulk purchase for sales promotions, premiums, fund-raising, and educational needs. Special books or book excerpts also can be created to fit specific needs. For details, write Putnam Special Markets, 375 Hudson Street, New York, NY 10014.

Avery
a member of
Penguin Putnam Inc.
375 Hudson Street
New York, NY 10014
www.penguinputnam.com

Library of Congress Cataloging-in-Publication Data

Phillips, Robert H.
Coping with endometriosis : sound, compassionate advice for alleviating the
physical and emotional symptoms of this frequently misunderstood
illness / Robert H. Phillips and Glenda Motta.
p.   cm.
Includes bibliographical references and index.
ISBN 1-58333-074-7
1. Endometriosis.   I. Motta, Glenda.   II. Title.
RG483.E53 P48   2000   00-042043
618.1—dc21

Printed in the United States of America

5   7   9   10   8   6   4

Book design by Jennifer Ann Daddio

This book is lovingly dedicated to my family—my wife, Sharon, and my three sons, Michael, Larry, and Steven; my daughter-in-law Donna and her family; my parents, sister, mother-in-law, nephews, niece, and favorite aunt; and all my other relatives and in-laws— and to my friends.

—R.H.P.

This book is dedicated with love and respect to my wonderful parents, especially my mom, who began suffering symptoms of endometriosis sixty years ago; to my friends Kathi, Becky, and Darlene, who gave me the courage to have surgery; and to my incredibly patient, quiet, understanding, and loving husband of twenty-nine years, Nick, who has always been understanding while I cope with endometriosis.

—G.J.M.

Contents

PART ONE

Endometriosis—An Overview

PART TWO

Your Emotions

PART THREE

Changes in General Lifestyle

PART FOUR

Interacting with Other People

PART FIVE
Living with Someone with Endometriosis

A Word About Gender

Your primary physician—as well as any other doctors who are involved in your treatment—may be male or female. To avoid using the awkward "he/she" when referring to any one healthcare provider, we use the female pronouns "she" and "her" in odd-numbered chapters and the male "he," "him," and "his" in the remaining chapters. This decision has been made in the interest of simplicity and clarity.

Preface

Endometriosis can have a major impact on you and your family. Certainly, there are many unknowns about this disease, its cause, and its treatment. But if you have questions, fears, or concerns, rest assured that you are not alone. Physicians or other healthcare professionals can answer some of your questions. You may find answers in other books or articles on the subject. There is also a wealth of information on the Internet. However, many questions still remain. Why? Experts just don't have all the answers, and this can be frustrating and upsetting. Even worse is the feeling of isolation you may experience, the feeling that you're alone because no one understands. This can really be depressing.

Medical science is making progress in finding the cause of endometriosis and developing new treatment options. But what about the psychological effects of endometriosis? A major factor in determining your potential to lead a normal, emotionally stable life is how well you cope with the strain of having this chronic illness.

Heavy stuff? You bet it is! But that's why this book was written. It is chock-full of information, suggestions, and strategies to help you, your doctor, your family, and your friends learn how to successfully cope with endometriosis.

The first part of the book presents basic information about the disease: what it is, how it is diagnosed, and what treatments are available. The remainder of the book deals with everyday challenges, including coping with emotions, making lifestyle changes, and living with others. We will explore each aspect in detail, examine many suggestions and strategies, and provide real-life examples. A lot of the information you'll be reading can—and does—apply to any chronic medical condition. This book, however, will focus specifically on your life with endometriosis.

As you learn to cope with endometriosis, it is important to realize that you are not alone; millions of other women or teenage girls and their families and friends are experiencing many of the same struggles and emotions. We hope that this is reassuring. Remember, though, that each person is unique, so symptoms will vary as can response to treatment. What works great for one may not work at all for another. Similarly, the psychological consequences of having endometriosis are quite unpredictable. Your life with endometriosis—the way it affects you and the way you react to it—will not be the same as anyone else's. Therefore, it will be up to *you* to use the suggestions and strategies presented in this book to help yourself cope as well as you possibly can. This book was written to help you take charge of your body and to become an active rather than a passive participant in your treatment plan.

Until such time as there is no longer a condition called endometriosis, you will have to learn to live with it. We hope this book will help both you and your family to do just that, and to do it comfortably and in control.

Robert H. Phillips, Ph.D.
Center for Coping
Hicksville, NY

Glenda J. Motta, R.N., M.P.H.
GM Associates, Inc.
Mitchellville, MD

Foreword

Endometriosis is one of the most prevalent gynecological disorders, affecting millions of women and girls around the world. The incidence of endometriosis diagnoses is on the rise, and we can no longer afford to treat the disease as an insignificant issue. Endometriosis can result in incapacitating pain, infertility, and repeated surgeries, and can render a woman or girl unable to go about her normal routine. This disease affects not only the patient, but also everyone around her.

However, there is hope.

Women everywhere are taking charge of their own healthcare, becoming empowered patients, and acting as partners in their disease diagnosis and treatment. Gone are the days when a patient will accept the "it's all in your head" diagnosis. Doctors and scientists are listening to the demand for more rapid diagnoses, more effective treatments, and ultimately, a cure for endometriosis. New research, particularly in the fields of Aromatase inhibitors, genetics, reproductive immunology, angiogenesis, environmental hazards, and diagnosis without invasive surgery, is particularly promising for the future. We have come a long way since Dr. Von Rokitansky first detailed the disease in 1860.

We have shattered the myths that pregnancy, hysterectomy, and menopause will cure the disease, and we are making great strides in earlier diagnoses at younger ages. We are also seeing an increase of physicians who are dedicating their practices to the diagnosis and expert treatment of endometriosis. These surgeons are specially trained to recognize the disease in all its manifestations and to eradicate endometriosis through minimally invasive means. We have seen advances by these surgeons in laparoscopic surgery, including microscopic laparoscopy and patient-assisted laparoscopy (PAL). These advances in surgery, coupled with scientific research, hold the key to unlocking the mysteries of endometriosis.

But we still don't have either an identified, singular cause of endometriosis or an absolute cure. Controversy, theories, and misconceptions abound. The endometriosis patient needs access to the most up-to-date, accurate educational information so she is able to make informed decisions about her treatment. Thanks to Glenda Motta, R.N., and Robert H. Phillips, Ph.D., endometriosis sufferers and their families have just that.

In *Coping with Endometriosis*, the authors provide a comprehensive, detailed review of the disease and its treatments, along with information on current forward-looking research, resources, and most important, coping strategies and hope for the future. Encompassing an overview of the disease, lifestyle changes, fertility, and sex and pregnancy, as well as strategies for coping with emotions, this detailed guide to life with endometriosis in an important tool in recovery. Educational, encouraging, and empowering, *Coping with Endometriosis* is one of the best guides and resources for all endometriosis sufferers and their families.

Michelle E. Marvel   Heather C. Guidone
Founder and Executive Director   Director of Operations
Endometriosis Research Center   Endometriosis Research Center

World Headquarters
630 Ibis Drive
Delray Beach, FL 33444
www.endocenter.org

PART ONE

Endometriosis—
an Overview

CHAPTER ONE

What Is Endometriosis?

Anne, a 26-year-old mother of one, had not been feeling well. She had been experiencing more and more pain, especially before and during her periods. Being shy, she didn't really want to mention this to anyone, but the pain was getting unbearable. She went to her gynecologist, expecting he'd tell her it was normal, though unpleasant, and give her some pills. Instead, after asking detailed questions and completing a physical and pelvic examination, the doctor asked her to sit down in his consultation room. Anne nervously approached the chair next to his desk and sat down. Her husband of five years sat by her side. The doctor looked at her and wasted no time in telling her, "Anne, I suspect you have endometriosis." Anne's immediate reaction was very similar to others who have been diagnosed with this disease. Trembling, she looked at the doctor and exclaimed, "What's endometriosis?"

What Is Endometriosis?

Endometriosis is a chronic disease of a woman's or teenage girl's reproductive and immune systems. Patches of endometrial tissue—similar to the tissue normally found only in the *endometrium*, the lining of the uterus—grow outside the uterus (the womb). This tissue develops into different types of "growths," also called "implants," "nodules," or "cysts," which can cause pain, bleeding, infertility, problems with your bowel or bladder, and many other symptoms or changes.

Fortunately, endometriosis is not contagious, and it is not a form of cancer. However, it is a serious disease that may cause chronic pain, disabling menstrual periods, and internal scarring. For some women, endometriosis can be extremely painful all the time. For others, the pain may be most severe during ovulation or before or during their menstrual period. Others may have very little or no pain.

To better understand this condition, let's discuss what happens during a normal menstrual cycle, and then how this relates to what happens in endometriosis.

WHAT HAPPENS DURING A NORMAL MENSTRUAL CYCLE?

Menstruation, a discharge of blood and tissue (from a nonpregnant uterus), normally occurs approximately every 28 days or so—from the time of puberty, when the reproductive organs become active, until menopause—except during pregnancy. During the monthly menstrual cycle, a thick, blood-rich cushion is prepared inside the uterus to protect and nourish a newly fertilized egg (which would mean you are pregnant). If an egg is not fertilized, it will not implant in this uterine lining, so it will not be needed. The blood and tissue of this lining, along with the unfertilized egg, are discharged from the body (menstruation), enabling this cycle to begin anew the following month.

The Menstrual Cycle in More Detail

Each month, some of the brain's hormones—the follicle-stimulating hormone (FSH), luteinizing hormone (LH), and gonadotrophin-releasing hormone (GnRH)—relay messages to your ovaries (the sex glands located on either side of your uterus). The ovaries then produce their own hormones: estrogen and progesterone. Follicle-stimulating hormone triggers the ripening of ovarian sacs (follicles), which contain the eggs. As the follicles grow, they secrete estrogen in greater amounts. The estrogen affects the lining of the uterus, signaling it to grow.

Only one of the follicles will mature fully, preparing to release an egg for possible fertilization. When this egg is mature, both progesterone and estrogen are secreted. These two hormones trigger the brain to release more hormones that then signal the follicle to release the egg.

At the middle point in the menstrual cycle, about the fourteenth day, ovulation occurs. The egg is discharged from the ovary. It travels through the fallopian tube to the uterus. At this stage, LH (luteinizing hormone) changes the follicle to the corpus luteum (a yellow mass). Now more progesterone than estrogen is secreted influencing the lining of the uterus to build up fluid and blood vessels to nourish the egg. The corpus luteum will continue to secrete hormones if the egg is fertilized to maintain the pregnancy.

If the egg is not fertilized, the corpus luteum degenerates and stops functioning. Progesterone production decreases, and the uterine lining, prepared to nourish a fertilized egg, cannot be maintained. This leads to menstruation (your period). Blood, tissue, and mucus from the lining, along with the remains of the egg, discharge from your body through the vaginal canal. It is like a tree shedding its leaves in the fall.

WHAT HAPPENS IN ENDOMETRIOSIS?

Although experts don't know for a fact what happens, the current belief is that, at times, all the menstrual debris is not eliminated during the monthly period. When a woman or teenage girl has endometriosis, this debris stays active and may travel to other sites. Cells implant in the ovaries, or the fallopian tubes, and may migrate to other body organs. Endometrial growths are most often found in the abdominal cavity—the area of the body containing the reproductive organs, as well as the bladder, small and large intestines, and kidneys. Endometriosis can attack any of these pelvic organs, the sides and walls of the pelvis, and the ligaments supporting the uterus. The most common area where endometriosis occurs is behind the uterus in the area known as the *cul-de-sac* or *pouch-of-Douglas.* Growths may also be found in the internal area between the vagina and rectum, on the outer surface of the uterus, on the intestines or in the rectum, on the bladder, vagina, cervix, and vulva (external genitals), or in abdominal surgery scars. In some circumstances, growths have been found outside the abdomen in the thigh, arm, lung, diaphragm and brain.

In endometriosis, endometrial tissue implanted outside the uterus behaves the way that endometrial tissue in the uterus normally does; the implants respond to monthly hormonal changes, swell, and become full of blood. At the end of every cycle, when hormonal changes cause the uterus to shed its lining in the menstrual flow, endometrial tissue growing outside the uterus also attempts to shed and so it, too, bleeds. But these cells and blood have nowhere to go. They have no way to leave the body as they would if they were in the uterus and were shed through the vaginal opening. Instead, the endometrial tissue produces its own estrogen and grows, building up month after month.

Initially, endometrial lesions may be so small that they can only be seen under a microscope. But they can grow to be as large as a grapefruit. The surrounding tissues may become inflamed or swollen, form scar tissue, and bleed even more. Any part of this process can impede normal organ function and can result in severe pain, infertility, and obstructions.

The Role of Prostaglandins

Menstrual pain and cramping is caused by an imbalance of prostaglandins—hormonelike substances that stimulate contractions of the uterus and other smooth muscles, like the bowel. When prostaglandins are released into the bloodstream as the endometrial lining breaks down, the uterus goes into spasm, resulting in cramping pain.

Women who have endometriosis tend to produce more prostaglandins than women who do not have it. Researchers think that this prostaglandin imbalance may cause many of the symptoms of endometriosis.

WHO GETS ENDOMETRIOSIS?

Endometriosis affects women and teenage girls of all races all over the world. Endometrial tissue has been found in autopsies of infants, premenstrual adolescents, posthysterectomy, and postmenopausal women (even in five men!) but generally occurs in women who are having menstrual periods. Experts don't know the exact numbers because so many cases remain undiagnosed. However, age at diagnosis ranges from the midteens to the forties. One study reported that more than 50% of teenage girls undergoing surgery for severe pelvic pain had lesions. The Endometriosis Association and the Endometriosis Research Center estimate that 2–4% of the general female population worldwide may have endometriosis. Endometriosis affects more women than breast cancer. The average delay from the beginning of symptoms to diagnosis of the disease is over nine years. The disease is often confused with pelvic inflammatory disease, bladder infections, irritable bowel syndrome, and a multitude of other conditions. This means millions of women and girls suffer needlessly and treatment is delayed.

Endometriosis was once considered a disease of "career-oriented" women. Because of this myth, many teenage girls and women may not be diagnosed with endometriosis for a long period of time. It was once believed that white women were at a higher risk for this disease than women of other races. As a result, nonwhite women are often misdiagnosed as having some other condition, when the true problem is endometriosis.

What Causes Endometriosis?

Why does endometriosis occur? Why do some women develop endometriosis while others do not? Why do endometrial cells migrate to other parts of the body? Unfortunately, the answers to these questions are not clear-cut, but as research continues we are beginning to understand the disease better.

Numerous risk factors seem to contribute to the development of endometriosis, the severity of the disease, variety of symptoms, and a woman's response to treatment. These include:

- Familial history—there seems to be a genetic predisposition for endometriosis.
- Women with higher estrogen levels and prolonged heavy menstrual periods are at an increased risk.
- Anatomic factors: cervical stenosis (a contraction of the narrow, lower end of the uterus that serves as a passageway between the uterus and vagina) increases risk. Your cervical opening must be wide enough for the menstrual debris and endometrial tissue to pass through each month. A too-narrow opening can interfere with this occurring.
- Exposure to environmental toxins, especially those that have an estrogenlike effect (see p.10).
- Lifestyle: low body weight and/or cigarette smoking reduces the risk by decreasing estrogen levels; diets high in estrogen level–increasing foods seem to increase risk. (One unproven theory is that fat stimulates excess estrogen production in the body, which stimulates endometriosis.)

- Contraceptives: using oral contraceptives may reduce progression of the disease.
- Obstetric history: some studies say that pregnancy and lactation (the period of weeks or months during which a child is nursed) reduces risk; other studies suggest that childlessness increases risk.

Despite the number of theories as to the cause of endometriosis, none seem to account for all cases. Let's look at some of the more commonly held theories currently being investigated.

THE RETROGRADE MENSTRUATION THEORY

Also called the transtubal migration theory, this view suggests that endometrial cells from the uterus flow backward through the fallopian tubes at the end of the cycle, finding their way into the abdomen where they implant and grow. Clearly, 90% of all women do *not* develop endometriosis, yet recent studies have shown that 90% of all women experience some retrograde menstruation. In most cases, when menstrual tissue debris flows outside of the uterus, it is destroyed before the tissue can implant, or seed. In women who develop endometriosis, however, the transplanted endometrial tissue somehow successfully seeds and grows. Eventually, the endometrial tissue develops its own blood supply and becomes an independent, growing mass.

THE EMBRYONIC TISSUE THEORY

According to this theory, endometriosis is a congenital condition in that endometrial tissue develops in the female embryo as the fetus grows. This theory suggests that some of the endometrial cells do not travel from the ducts that become the lining of the uterus but stay in the pelvic cavity. When a young girl begins puberty and hormones are produced, this displaced tissue starts producing the symptoms typical of endometriosis. This might explain why some girls have severe pain as soon as they start their menstrual periods.

THE GENETIC THEORY

Endometriosis often runs in families. Some studies indicate that women with endometriosis often come from families where others have the disease—primarily mothers and sisters—and are much more likely to have daughters with the disease. Studies suggest that there is a sevenfold increase in the risk of endometriosis in mothers and sisters of women with endometriosis. Scientists believe that genetic susceptibility may play a role, to a degree that depends on personal factors and, perhaps, environmental stimuli. The Oxford Endometriosis Gene (OXEGENE) study, a worldwide research study based at the Oxford University, is seeking to isolate the specific gene(s) to prove the hereditary connections.

THE LYMPHATIC DISTRIBUTION THEORY

Remember that the endometrial tissue growing outside of the uterus eventually develops its own blood supply and becomes an independent, growing mass. This theory suggests that, in ways similar to the spread of a tumor, a piece of the implanted tissue may break off from the primary site, enter a blood or lymph vessel, and spread to distant body sites. As these free-floating pieces of endometrial tissue implant, grow, and develop their own blood supply, the process repeats itself. This theory is supported by the fact that endometrial implants have been found as far away as the lungs, legs, groin, and brain.

IMMUNE SYSTEM THEORIES

If retrograde menstruation is common among most women, why would some women develop endometriosis while others do not? The answer to this question may lie in the differences in immune system functioning of women with and without the disease. Current studies clearly indicate that the immune system plays a role in endometriosis and that women with endometriosis have immune system abnormalities.

Normally, your immune system protects you by generating cells that fight the invasion of germs and other foreign bodies. Cells called antibodies attack the foreign invaders. One immune system theory suggests that endometrial cells misplaced in the peritoneal cavity are recognized as "foreign" by the local immune cells. In women who have healthy immune systems, endometrial cells that migrate to other locations are destroyed. This theory suggests that if you have endometriosis, the immune system's antibodies seem less able to eliminate this misplaced tissue, which then grows into endometriosis.

Other studies strongly suggest that endometriosis should be classified as an autoimmune disease, a condition in which the antibodies of the body's immune system for some reason turn around and fight healthy tissue within the body. This is also supported by the fact that women with endometriosis typically suffer from other autoimmune conditions, including chronic fatigue, lupus, rheumatoid arthritis, psoriasis, ulcerative colitis, multiple sclerosis, and chronic yeast infections (candida).

ENVIRONMENTAL POLLUTANTS

Recent studies have also explored the role of environmental factors as contributors to the development of endometriosis. Research suggests that environmental toxins, such as dioxin and PCBs (polychlorinated biphenyls), are linked to endometriosis. The Environmental Protection Agency has identified that one effect of dioxin is a "higher probability of experiencing endometriosis and the reduced ability to withstand an immunoloical challenge." Dioxin is present in trace amounts in the entire range of chlorine-bleached paper products, such as sanitary napkins and tampons, toilet paper, facial tissues, disposable diapers, paper plates and towels, coffee filters and cigarette papers. The most common source of dioxin comes from food contaminated by pesticides. PCBs are compounds that were widely used as electrical insulators, in carbonless paper, specialty inks, and paints, and as additives in plastics. Waste water from the manufacture of these products and from sewage treatment plants that process the waste have contaminated our water and soil. PCBs last a very long time. They were banned in the United States and Canada by 1980 but still remain in our environment.

Studies have investigated the profound effects of *xenoestrogens* (foreign substances originating outside the body that mimic the action of estrogen) on hormone balance. Nearly all of these are petrochemically based, that is, they are derived from petroleum oil. Machines are run on petroleum fuels; buildings are heated with petroleum oil; millions of products, including plastics, microchips, medicines, personal care products, clothing, food, soaps, pesticides, herbicides, and even perfumes, are made from petrochemicals or contain them. These environmental petrochemicals mimic and/or interfere with female and male hormones and adversely affect development and reproduction in animal wildlife. To date, studies have been inconclusive as to whether this exposure could cause endometriosis. However, researchers speculate that our petrochemical age has spawned diseases unknown before the present age, and that endometriosis is one of them.

DELAYED CHILDBEARING

Women who delay childbearing were historically thought to be at higher risk for endometriosis. In fact, endometriosis used to be called the "career woman's disease," referring to women who put off pregnancy. This myth was perpetuated by uninformed physicians and reinforced by a lack of research. In fact, recent studies show there is no difference in the incidence of endometriosis among women who have been pregnant and those who have not. Some women are still mistakenly told that if they have a baby, the disease will be cured. The truth is, since the hormones made by the placenta during pregnancy prevent ovulation, the progression of endometriosis may be reduced or stopped during pregnancy. However, researchers conclude that pregnancy offers no protection against having endometriosis.

Although it is unfortunate that the actual causes of endometriosis have not yet been determined, there are certain treatments that can markedly reduce the impact the disease has on your body. (More about this later.) Hopefully, research will provide more insight into the causes of endometriosis, which can lead to a cure.

What Are the Symptoms of Endometriosis?

The symptoms of endometriosis vary tremendously from person to person. Some women exhibit many symptoms, while others have only a few or even none at all.

Often symptoms are unpredictable and can be easily confused with those of other diseases. It is not unusual for young women with endometriosis to misconstrue elements of the disease as normal menstrual symptoms. Many women escape proper diagnosis and continue to suffer, believing this is normal.

For the most part the symptoms of endometriosis can be divided into the following main categories: pain, fatigue, bowel and bladder complications, heavy or irregular bleeding, and fertility problems.

PAIN

Pain is, by far, the most common symptom! It is estimated that at least 90% of all women with endometriosis experience pelvic pain. In a recent survey of four thousand women tabulated by the Endometriosis Association, 96% experienced pain—95% at the time of the menstrual period, 83% at the time of ovulation, and 75% at other times as well. The degree of pain can range from mild to severe, and need not be directly related to the severity of the disease. Pain is often an indication of where, and to what extent, the endometrial lesions are growing.

Pain may occur as a result of any of the following:

- Inflammation (caused by endometrial implants secreting irritating substances, such as histamines).
- The presence of scar tissue or adhesions. (Adhesions are fibrous bands that form as a result of the inflammatory process that occurs with endometriosis. They "glue" together surfaces and organs that are normally separate, potentially interfering with their mobility and function.)
- Leaking endometrial growths release inflammatory substances.
- Compression or blockage of other abdominal organs (such as the bowel or ureters—the tubes that carry urine from the kidneys to the bladder).
- Compression of endometrial nodules deep in the pelvis.
- Endometrial invasion of the urinary tract (including the bladder or ureters).
- Endometrial invasion of the gastrointestinal tract (the small bowel or large intestine).

The most common types of pain are:

- **Pelvic pain.** It can occur in one pelvic organ, such as an ovary or the uterus, in several pelvic organs, or throughout the pelvis, and often involves cramps and bloating. Pelvic pain can occur both with, and prior to, menstruation and can occur with ovulation. Pain with ovulation has been reported to be very high among women whose pelvic symptoms started before age 20.

- **Menstrual pain.** Continuous pain before and through menstruation can actually serve as a good diagnostic sign of endometriosis. Severe menstrual cramps, called dysmenorrhea, felt in both the abdomen or lower back may be accompanied by dizziness and headaches. Women who have endometriosis and severe menstrual cramps have what is called secondary *dysmenorrhea*, which means that the pain is caused by the disease.

- **Painful sex.** Women with endometriosis often experience pain during sexual activities, About two-thirds of women with endometriosis report pain that continues even after intercourse, a condition known as dyspareunia. The most common area for endometriosis to occur is behind the uterus in the cul-de-sac, or pouch-of-Douglas. If lesions in this area push the uterus into a tilted-back position (called retroversion), deep vaginal penetration during sexual intercourse can move the uterus around or pull it out of its normal position, causing extreme pain. The pain may be worse if you have intercourse during your menstrual period when the endometrial implants are swollen and bleeding. Bleeding often continues after intercourse because the thrust of the penis bruises or damages the endometrial implants.

- **Pain with bowel movements.** Lesions in the area between the uterus and the rectum can cause rectal pressure and pain with bowel movements. In fact, 85% of women with endometriosis experience nausea, vomiting, upset stomach, diarrhea, painful bowel movements, bloating, or other intestinal distress during their period.

Because implants on or near the bowel produce chronic gastro-intestinal symptoms, endometriosis can be confused with irritable bowel syndrome or spastic colon. You may have gastrointestinal symptoms caused by other factors, including yeast (candida), the release of prostaglandins, endometriosis on the cul-de-sac irritating the bowel, or an imbalance in bacterial flora in the intestine.

FATIGUE

The second most common symptom of endometriosis is fatigue, low energy, or exhaustion. According to a study by the Endometriosis Association, 87% of women with endometriosis experience fatigue. Unfortunately, fatigue is a vague symptom and is often dismissed by physicians as unimportant. If you suffer from endometriosis, you might find that the bed is your favorite place for a few days each month during your period. Many women discover their energy levels are unpredictable . You may wake in the morning feeling fine and experience fatigue that comes on quickly during the day. On the other hand, you may awaken in the morning feeling completely exhausted and find that your energy level builds during the day.

BOWEL AND BLADDER COMPLICATIONS

Rectal bleeding and blood in the stool is not uncommon but should be investigated, and other bowel problems, such as polyps, should be ruled out.

Endometriosis can also attach to, push on, or invade the ureters or the bladder, causing symptoms that mimic urinary tract infection—frequent or painful urination, urinary retention, blood in the urine during menstruation, or flank pain (along the side of the body between the ribs and hips).

A disease known as interstitial cystitis (IC), sometimes associated with endometriosis, is a chronic inflammation of the bladder wall that occurs even though there are no bacteria or infections present. The most common symptoms of IC include a frequent or urgent need to urinate; pain in the bladder, urethra, or vagina; pain relieved by voiding; pain with sex; difficulty emptying the bladder; and difficulty starting urine flow. Bladder endometriosis may be mistaken for IC, so it is important that the exact cause of your symptoms be found and treated whenever possible.

HEAVY OR IRREGULAR BLEEDING

About two-thirds of women with endometriosis experience heavy, irregular, or abnormal bleeding known as menorrhagia. Some women have such a heavy flow during their periods that they routinely bleed through one or two tampons and a pad even into the second or third day of their period. Others experience bleeding in between normal periods, a condition known as dysfunctional uterine bleeding (DUB). Menorrhagia and DUB can also be caused by thyroid problems or fibroids, so these should be ruled out before a diagnosis of endometriosis is confirmed.

FERTILITY PROBLEMS

Endometriosis is a major factor that contributes to infertility. Some studies estimate that 30% to 40% of women with endometriosis are infertile. This is two to three times the rate of infertility in the general population. About 50% of women with unexplained infertility are found to have endometriosis when a laparoscopy (a procedure that uses a scope to examine the reproductive organs) is performed. Endometrial lesions can cause scarring and adhesions that prevent ovulation or block the passage of eggs through the fallopian tubes. If fertilization does occur, endometriosis may interfere with normal implantation and growth of the fertilized egg.

OTHER SYMPTOMS

In addition to the symptoms already mentioned, women with endometriosis can experience dizziness, migraine headaches, low back pain, poor resistance to infections, extensive allergies, chemical sensitivities, vaginal discharge between periods, yeast infections, and low-grade fever.

WHEN DO SYMPTOMS OCCUR?

Many women experience a variety of symptoms throughout their menstrual cycles. Ovulation is painful for most women. The severity of symptoms may coincide with fluctuations of estrogen and progesterone levels in the body. It is very important to be aware of your body so you can identify changes or new symptoms as they occur. Any symptom you experience regularly during your cycle should be reported to your doctor, especially those related to bowel habits, rectal bleeding, pain with sex, problems urinating, or severe menstrual cramps.

How Is Endometriosis Diagnosed?

Endometriosis is not a difficult disease to diagnosis. Unfortunately, diagnosis is often delayed in spite of symptoms. Too many physicians don't take menstrual pain seriously in young girls—and even in women! Others may confuse endometriosis with conditions such as pelvic inflammatory disease, premenstrual syndrome, or inflammation of reproductive organs. Another reason for the delay in diagnosis is that many women believe that pain with the menstrual cycle is normal and so they don't report their symptoms to their doctor. Many women have never heard of endometriosis and so don't associate their pain with a disease.

Myths about women's reproductive cycles continue to exist. Often young girls and women believe—or are told by physicians—that "the pain is all in your head." Or maybe their mothers told them to "grin and bear it." Remember that severe pain is not normal, so take control of your health and your medical treatment. Play an active rather than a passive role. Gather information, ask questions, and seek a second or even third opinion if you have to.

Sometimes endometrial growths can be felt during pelvic examination. A definitive diagnosis of endometriosis is made after careful consideration of your medical history, a physical examination, and an "internal exploration," using a minor surgical procedure called laparoscopy.

There are several blood tests that may be used to try to diagnose endometriosis. One is the hemoglobin level, a test for anemia. However, anemia occurs with many other conditions, not just endometriosis. Another is CA125, a blood test for a cell surface protein found in pelvic organs. However, at this time there is no blood test that specifically detects endometriosis, although current research is attempting to develop one.

Other diagnostic tests, such as ultrasound scans and x-rays, may be useful. Pelvic ultrasounds are limited because they may not detect minor forms of endometriosis (which can cause severe pain). There are no x-rays that specifically show endometriosis, but the tubal x-ray (hysterosalpingogram) may give some clues to tubal occlusion. You might need specialized x-rays if your endometriosis involves other body organs, such as the bowel.

Occasionally, woman are diagnosed with endometriosis during surgery for what was thought to be acute appendicitis, gallbladder disease, or cancer. Acute abdominal pain may result in exploratory surgery and a discovery of endometriosis. Or women who undergo laparoscopy for infertility may be diagnosed.

MEDICAL HISTORY

The first step in the diagnostic process is obtaining a detailed medical history. Here are some questions the doctor might ask:

- What symptoms are you experiencing (When do they occur? How long do they last?)
- What makes your symptoms worse or better?
- How would you describe your menstrual pain, pain with sex, or other pain?
- Does the pain come and go?
- Does the pain interfere with your personal routine, such as eating, getting dressed, intercourse, and so on?
- Do you have other symptoms besides menstrual cramps, such as periodic changes in bowel habits or problems with urination?
- Is there any family history of illness (especially endometriosis, if suspected)?
- Has there been any difficulty conceiving? Is there any family history of infertility? Is there any history of miscarriages?

PHYSICAL EXAMINATION

After taking your medical history, your doctor will give you a complete physical exam, including a pelvic exam. She will be checking for endometrial implants or nodules, areas of tenderness or thickening in your pelvis, as well as evidence of retroversion, or tilting-backward, of your uterus.

Your physician will do an examination using both hands, inserting one or two fingers of one hand into your vagina to push up on the uterus behind the cervix, while at the same time sweeping the other hand down your lower abdomen, beginning at the belly button. In this way, the doctor can feel the uterus, ovaries, and the areas surrounding these internal organs between two hands. Then the doctor will do a recto-vaginal exam, inserting an index finger into the vagina while inserting a middle finger into the rectum, to feel behind the uterus. The doctor can feel ovarian cysts and even rectal abnormalities during this part of the exam that could otherwise be missed.

TAKING A LOOK "INSIDE"

Regardless of the information obtained during the history and physical examination, a diagnosis of endometriosis can not be definitive without the doctor seeing signs of endometrial growths. In order to do this, a procedure known as a laparoscopy is necessary. This is a minor surgical procedure, usually done on an outpatient basis. After general anesthesia is administered, a small key-hole incision is made in or near the belly button. Carbon dioxide gas is introduced to the abdomen to inflate it. A lighted tube called a laparoscope is inserted through the incision into the abdomen so the doctor can "visualize," or see, the pelvic cavity and the organs contained there.

During the laproscopy, the doctor can identify the number, size, and location of endometrial growths or implants. Endometrial growths can have many appearances: the classic "powder-burn" or "blueberry" lesion; white lesions that mimic scar tissue; "chocolate cysts," so-called because of the color of the old blood inside the cyst; clear, slightly brown, or yellow blue-colored lesions, "strawberry," or flamelike, lesions; pockets in the peritoneal cavity; and deep nodules in the cul-de-sac.

The doctor may also remove some tissue and send it for a biopsy (microscopic examination in the laboratory) to confirm the diagnosis. On other occasions, the doctor will remove endometrial growths, as part of the treatment, during the laparoscopy. When finished, the gas is released and your incision is closed with stitches.

Sometimes, doctors may detect endometrial growths using other types of "scope" procedures, such as a cystoscopy (to see inside the bladder), a sigmoidoscopy (to see inside the rectum), or a colonoscopy (to see further into the large intestine than sigmoidoscopy permits). Less often, a major abdominal surgical procedure called laparotomy may be used for diagnostic and treatment purposes. See chapter 2 for a more complete description of these procedures.

Newer technology, such as nuclear imaging, Doppler color, and MRI (magnetic resonance imaging), provide methods to reveal anatomically displaced cells or tissues by external scanning. Now used to detect tumors and sites of infection, these imaging techniques may offer more accurate and less invasive ways to diagnose endometriosis.

A new procedure called microlaparoscopy can be used in the office under local or light sedation to evaluate the pelvis, see the extent of endometriosis, and excise easily accessible lesions. A laparoscope the size of a needle is used, and no sutures are required. The small scope allows you to remain awake so the surgeon can touch an implant and ask you if that is where the pain is.

STAGES OF ENDOMETRIOSIS

Endometriosis is classified into stages, indicating the degree to which it is affecting other organs. Classification is based on the location of implants, whether the endometriosis is superficial or deep, and if there are adhesions present.

The stage is determined by a weighted point system. During an examination of the pelvis, your physician notes the number, size, and location of endometrial implants, endometriomas (masses that contain endometrial tissue), and adhesions. The severity of the endometriosis or adhesions located in the peritoneum, on the ovaries, the fallopian tubes, and the cul-de-sac is assigned a score, and the total determines the stage.

There are four stages of endometriosis. Stage I is minimal. Endometriosis in the peritoneum (the abdominal cavity) is superficial, and only one ovary is involved. The endometrial lesions are small and not widespread. Stage II is mild. There is deep endometriosis in the peritoneum and both ovaries have superficial involvement. Stage III is moderate. There can be superficial or deep endometriosis in the peritoneum. The cul-de-sac (the area between the wall of the uterus and the rectum) is involved. Lesions are deep in one ovary, and the fallopian tubes are often affected. Adhesions are deep. Stage IV is severe. The number and type of implants are large; there are dense adhesions in the peritoneum, the fallopian tubes, and the ovaries. Often, there is extensive scar tissue. There is considerable disease in many locations such as the ovaries, fallopian tubes, bladder, bowel, appendix, peritoneum, and cul-de-sac.

The staging system was revised in 1996 and is available from the American Society for Reproductive Medicine. It is flawed in that the staging is not related to pain. (In some women, lesions may be small but cause severe pain. Others may have large lesions without a lot of pain.) It also does not label the changes that may be going on in the immune system and does not allow for the fact that implants may fluctuate in size.

How Serious Is Endometriosis?

While any chronic disease can be serious, this does not necessarily mean that you will develop a serious case. Endometriosis ranges from mild to severe, depending on which organs are affected by growths, the degree to which they're affected, and other symptoms.

For example, the severity of endometriosis can be better measured by the intensity of your pain. Does it interfere with your ability to work? Does it make sex painful? Does it interfere with conception? If you use appropriate health procedures to take care of yourself properly, follow a well-structured treatment plan, and keep in close contact with your physician, you can increase the chances of endometriosis having a milder impact on your quality of life.

What Is the Prognosis?

Endometriosis is a chronic disease with no cure at the present time, which means that it can last as long as you are alive. New data from the world's largest research registry on endometriosis show that women with endometriosis and their families have a heightened risk of breast cancer, melanoma, and ovarian cancer. There is also a greater risk of non-Hodgkins lymphoma in these families and a significantly higher incidence of diabetes, thyroid disorders, and other autoimmune diseases such as rheumatoid arthritis, lupus, multiple sclerosis, and Ménière's disease.

Despite the fact that treatment for endometriosis is becoming more successful, it is impossible to predict the future course of the disease. There is no pattern. Serious problems with endometriosis occur when it has a destructive affect on important internal organs. Early diagnosis and aggressive treatment is critical because it does not improve if ignored.

Medical advances have been able to provide better management, so many women can now live long, reasonably normal lives. However, some women cannot totally escape the pain, which, despite treatment, may continue to range from mild to debilitating. In order to best live with endometriosis, it is essential to go beyond the medical treatment and do everything you can to deal with the pain and emotional stress.

CHAPTER TWO

How Is Endometriosis Treated?

So far, we have discussed what endometriosis is, who may get it, some of the symptoms, and how it is diagnosed, as well as other details about the disease. Terrific—but you're probably less concerned about what it is and where it came from than you are about feeling better. True? You probably have some important questions, such as: What can your doctor do for you? What can you do for yourself? What are the different treatments for endometriosis, and how can they help you? How do you control your symptoms? How can you help yourself get back into the mainstream of life? Let's begin by answering some of these questions.

Each Person Is Unique

Your endometriosis symptoms are unique and may be very different from other women you know, meet, or even read about. So your treatment program will be unique as well, and specific to your own needs.

On the basis of experience, every physician will have varying opinions about which approaches may work best. A lot of trial and error will go into developing the best treatment plan for you, and you may feel like a human guinea pig. But remember, this is only because the goal is to find the treatment protocol that works best for you.

It is very important for you to feel at ease with your physician. You want to have confidence that the prescribed interventions will work. What if you heard that somebody else with endometriosis was following a different program prescribed by another physician, and you started to believe that it was working better than yours? You might start losing confidence in your treatment plan, and then in your own physician. Not a great feeling, is it? Remember, there is no one answer! What works for other women will not necessarily work for you.

In general, treatment can vary, depending on age; the severity of the disease; the extent of the bleeding, pain, and other symptoms; lifestyle; and personal preference. A carefully structured, comprehensive treatment program can be successful in controlling symptoms to the point where they no longer interrupt normal activity. However, there are times when some or all of the approaches are not 100% successful or are not able to reduce all of your symptoms. Medications or other treatments may not adequately control your endometriosis, or complications may arise. But you'll work with your physician, and you'll cross that bridge if and when you come to it.

So what should you do? Make sure you're seeing a doctor or other health-care professional you can trust, then work closely with him. (To learn more about this, see Chapter 21.) Because you might receive various forms of treatment at different times, it is important to be aware of all the available options. Make sure you fully understand your doctor's recommendation and the reason for it. Depending on your individual condition, you may or may not be able to consider different options. If your situation *does* allow you to make a choice, you should be as informed as possible to make the best decision. There are many ways to obtain facts to guide your decision-making. Obviously, one way is to read this book. Other ways include contacting the Endometriosis Association and the Endometriosis Research Center, getting information from reliable sources on the Internet, and talking to other women who have this disease. Once you feel that you understand your physician's treatment choice, consider getting a second opinion—and a third, if necessary. Make sure that you're getting the best, most appropriate, and potentially helpful treatment possible. (See chapter 21 for more information on second opinions.)

What Are the Goals of Treatment?

The ideal outcome would, of course, be a cure, in which endometrial lesions—or at least endometriosis symptoms—no longer exist. Because there is no known cure for endometriosis, treatment ideally aims at a suppression of symptoms. You want to feel better, right? Well, that's the primary intent of treatment, along with protecting and strengthening your body. Experts believe that women with endometriosis do best following a comprehensive treatment program that enhances the effectiveness of their immune system, while determining what they need to change about their lives. Most important, you must develop a greater understanding of what is needed for true healing, not just for masking your physical symptoms.

You want to reduce the impact of your symptoms. However, the ideal outcome is remission, when symptoms no longer exist or are at least under control and you can function at a maximum level. Adjusting your general lifestyle, changing your behavior and activities, and learning to cope with the many emotional reactions you may be experiencing can be very helpful.

There are five specific goals for treatment of endometriosis.

- To control the disease by preventing the development of new lesions.
- To stop the progression of existing lesions.
- To maintain or restore fertility for those women trying to conceive by eliminating any endometrial-related obstacles to conception. (More about this in chapter 23.)
- To treat immune factors linked to endometriosis
- To increase comfort by alleviating pain and other symptoms that disrupt your lifestyle.

What Are the Components of Treatment Programs?

All treatment programs should involve a number of components, including the surgical or prescribed medical treatment as well as a comprehensive regimen of stress management, exercise, nutrition, and psychological improvement. In addition, many women find relief from complementary or alternative strategies. This chapter provides an overview of these different components. More details, such as information on medications specifically prescribed for pain, are given later.

MEDICAL TREATMENT

There are two main categories of medical treatment for endometriosis: medication and surgery. Although these categories are distinctly different and can be used separately, in many cases they are used in combination. For example, many surgical treatments are followed by the use of medication to help stop the development of new growths or to shrink existing ones. Endometriosis has an underlying immune system component, which means women often have a complex of other symptoms, including chronic fatigue, nausea, bowel problems, flulike symptoms, headaches, and PMS. Immune treatment should be considered along with medical or surgical interventions. This involves identifying possible allergens and infections, such as candida albicans (yeast). Treatment includes desensitization, neutralization, and tolerization for allergy symptoms that do not respond to medications, improving immune function throughout, and stress reduction.

Prescribed medications will vary, depending on the therapeutic goal. Certain medications are prescribed to shrink or prevent the growth of implants and adhesions, while others are appropriate if the primary goal is to reduce pain. If the major concern is to enhance fertility, the treatment course may be altogether different.

Medication (Hormonal Treatment)

Many of the current medical treatments for endometriosis attempt to control estrogen production, which causes endometrial tissue to grow. Researchers have discovered that both pregnancy and menopause may result in shrinkage of endometrial growths. Current medications used for endometriosis stop ovulation or suppress the release of estrogen from the ovaries. As a result, endometrial tissue growth slows down or stops, and previously formed growths may "dry up." Hormonal drugs are used to create a "pseudomenopause" or a "pseudopregnancy," stopping ovulation for as long a time as possible. This is called suppressive medical treatment. It does *not* cure endometriosis but hopefully reduces the inflammation in lesions and leads to a period of remission or at least reduced pain.

Some women experience immediate and substantial relief from hormonal medications used either alone or in conjunction with surgery. However, in some cases, unfortunately, once hormone treatment stops, endometrial growths return to their original size and pain becomes even worse than before.

Several different types of hormonal regimens are prescribed for endometriosis. They include a testosterone derivative (danazol); GnRH, (gonadotropin-releasing hormones), oral contraceptives or birth control pills (a combination of estrogen and progesterone); and progestogens alone. Let's discuss each of these main types in more detail.

Danazol. The first drug approved by the Food and Drug Administration (FDA) specifically for the treatment of endometriosis, danazol has been widely used for many years. It is commonly marketed under the brand name Danocrine. It is a synthetic male hormone derivative that works to reduce the size of existing endometrial lesions, prevent the growth of new implants, and relieve pain. It does this in two different ways. First, it acts as an *antiestrogen* drug, which means it opposes the role of estrogen in the body. Danazol prevents the pituitary gland from producing and releasing LH and FSH, the hormones necessary for ovulation. Using danazol puts a woman's body in a pseudomenopausal state, by preventing ovulation and menstruation.

Second, danazol is an *immunosuppressant* agent, which means it inhibits the formation of antibodies. The hope is that taking danazol will reduce the number of cells that fight against the endometrial tissue and interrupting the pattern of inflammation and infertility.

Some 80% or more of women on danazol find that it reduces endometriosis symptoms. Treatment with danazol results in immediate pain relief in up to 95% of women, although recurrence of symptoms after discontinuation is common.

A woman who takes danazol should start the drug during her period, when pregnancy is ruled out. Therapy should continue uninterrupted for three to six months, but no longer. Experience with long-term therapy is limited, and some potentially life-threatening complications, such as intraabdominal hemorrhage and increased intracranial pressure (pressure in the skull that causes stroke and vision problems), have been reported. Some women experience serious side effects after being on danazol for only a short time. So it is important to report any problems to your physician.

There can be adverse effects with Danazol. These include:

- **Side effects.** Danazol acts like the androgenic (male) sex hormone, testosterone. The common adverse effects experienced by 30–50% of women include acne, decreased sex drive, headaches, hot flashes, oily skin and hair, reduction in breast size, and weight gain. Problems, experienced by 15–25% of women, include bloating and fluid retention, abnormal facial and body hair growth, emotional instability, depression, nervousness, fatigue, muscle cramps, and vaginal dryness and irritation. Less frequently reported problems include breast pain, deepening of the voice, insomnia, nausea, rash, visual disturbances, and hair loss. Liver enzymes may also become abnormal while a woman is taking danazol, and they should be checked every six weeks. Fortunately, most of these symptoms are reversible when treatment is stopped, although a few may not be, such as loss of frontal hair and deepening of the voice.

- **Recurrence of endometriosis.** More than a third of women using danazol will experience a recurrence of endometriosis within three years. Between 30 and 60% of women experience gradual return of pain within one year after treatment; for 20%, symptoms will require further therapy. Unlike the GnRH drugs, danazol has not been limited by regulatory authorities to one course of treatment.

- **Birth defects.** Danazol is considered unsafe if there is any chance that a woman is pregnant, because of the significant risk of abnormal fetal development. Women taking danazol should consistently use an effective barrier form of birth control (eg., diaphragm, condom) to prevent pregnancy.

GnRH Agonists. Approved by the FDA for the treatment of endometriosis in 1990, the GnRH agonists have subsequently become a first-choice treatment for pain. Gonadotropin-releasing hormones are commonly marketed under the names Synarel (naferalin acetate), a nasal spray; Lupron (leuprolide acetate), an intramuscular injection; and Zoladex (goserelin acetate), administered as an implant placed under the skin into the abdominal wall. All forms seem to be equally effective.

Under the influence of these drugs, endometrial lesions tend to shrink in size. If given continuously, they stimulate, then paradoxically suppress natural hormones, in many cases, effectively reducing pain.

As with danazol, these drugs block the pituitary gland from producing FSH and LH, the hormones that lead to the production of estrogen, inducing a pseudomenopausal state. This type of aggressive medical intervention is used to lower estrogen levels in the body, which then reduces growth of endometrial lesions.

Treatment typically lasts for six months. The main difference between the various GnRH agonists is their dosage and form. They can be given by injection into a muscle, implanted below the skin, or self-administered as an intranasal spray. After a course of GnRH agonists, switching to birth control pills or progestogens can often prolong the relief from pain for some women.

Clinical studies show both GnRH and danazol therapy produce similar levels of pain relief. The recurrence rate of endometriosis after treatment with GnRH appears to be similar to that of other medical therapies. In addition, there is no difference in the effect on fertility after taking one drug over another. Remember, both danazol and GnRH drugs can have multiple adverse side effects and treatment provides only a temporary suppression of endometriosis. Discuss your options thoroughly with your doctor and work together to select which medication best fits into your overall treatment program.

Like danazol, there can be problems with GnRH agonists. These include:

- **Side effects.** GnRH agonists produce menopause-like side effects, such as hot flashes and bone demineralization, vaginal dryness, headaches, depression, decreased sex drive, breast reduction, insomnia, increases in "bad" cholesterol (LDL) and decreases in "good" cholesterol (HDL), and an increased risk of cardiovascular disease. Weakening of the bones is the most serious of these side effects, and a hormone replacement regimen is usually prescribed at the same time. Unfortunately, since there are no conclusive studies showing this supplementation regimen works, women who select treatment with a GnRH agonist should have bone density studies performed before beginning the treatment.

- **Short-term usage.** Because of the serious side effects of GnRH agonists, they are only approved for six months. Often, they are used to shrink growths before surgery or while trying to conceive. Before starting treatment, your doctor should make absolutely sure you are not pregnant because the drugs may cause harm to the developing fetus. Although it is unlikely, it is possible to become pregnant when taking GnRH agonists. Make sure you use a barrier method of contraception during treatment.

- **Recurrence of endometriosis.** The recurrence rate of endometrial lesions after cessation of GnRH treatment ranges from 25% for women with minimal disease to approximately 70% in women with severe disease. Be sure to carefully weigh the short-term relief against potential long-term risks with your doctor.

- **Varying effectiveness.** For some women, GnRH agonists work very well. For others there may be minimal, if any, positive effects.

Birth Control Pills. Oral contraceptives, or birth control pills, are sometimes prescribed as treatment for mild cases of endometriosis. They are marketed under many different names. They can be taken orally or by injection to create a pseudopregnancy. The pills that are most often prescribed are those with a high ratio of progesterone to estrogen. Oral contraceptives prescribed for endometriosis symptoms can be prescribed to be taken cyclically (the woman will have a monthly period) or continuously (the woman will not have a monthly period during treatment).

Oral contraceptives are most commonly prescribed to treat minor endometriosis pain, and some studies have shown that they provide pain relief for 75% or more of the women who take them. There are few studies regarding their effect on endometrial implants.

In some cases, these hormones may even worsen symptoms. Many physicians question the use of pills containing estrogen, since it is known to stimulate endometriosis. As a result, contraceptives continue to be controversial.

The side effects of contraceptive hormones can include nausea, high blood pressure, blood clots, enlargement of the uterus, weight gain, mood swings, and headaches.

Progestogens. These substances act like progesterone, a sex hormone. There are a large number of progestogens, ranging from synthetically produced chemicals (called progestins) to derivatives of male hormones. Progestins (the synthetically produced progestogens) are marketed under names such as Provera (medroxyprogesterone acetate tablets) and DepoProvera (medroxyprogesterone acetate injection).

Progestins inhibit the effects of estrogen on endometrial tissue, resulting in shrinkage of the implants. They must be taken in high doses to achieve any positive results, and side effects vary greatly, depending on the specific progestogen, the dosage, the interval of treatment, and the route of administration. Because they mimic pregnancy, these drugs usually lighten or stop periods. Common side effects include bleeding between periods, nausea, breast tenderness, fluid retention, headache, weight gain, and depression. Taking synthetic progestogens decreases your body's natural level of the hormone progesterone, so you may have more severe premenstrual syndrome. Progestogens do not seem to improve fertility.

Another option in this category is natural progesterone, which is identical to the hormone the body normally produces. Some women with endometriosis have a high blood level of estrogen and a relatively low blood level of progesterone, the hormone that works to balance excess estrogen. Over time, natural progesterone helps rebalance the estrogen–progesterone ratio and decreases the size of endometrial lesions.

One of the main advantages of natural progesterone is that no serious or irreversible side effects are reported from its use. Some women do have minor reactions as their bodies adjust to it, such as drowsiness, breast tenderness, water retention, spotting, or a skin reaction to the cream.

Natural progesterone is available in oral tablets, skin cream, oils, or under-the-tongue drops. Transdermal natural progesterone (the type applied to the skin) has an advantage over tablets because much lower amounts are required for therapeutic effect. A small number of users have reported an allergic skin reaction to the cream. Usually, doctors recommend two ounces of cream per month, applied to soft areas of the skin, such as the face, neck, and abdomen, on days 10 to 28 of the menstrual cycle. Another choice is natural progesterone capsules taken orally each day, also taken on days 10 to 28 of each cycle.

Since manufacturers of natural progesterone are restricted by the FDA from labeling their products with directions for use, ask your doctor to tailor an individual program. In addition, be sure to research for a reputable source.

New Drugs. Researchers are constantly investigating new medications to treat endometriosis. One example is an antiestrogen drug, raloxifene, that seems to be effective in reducing hot flashes and bone demineralization without causing endometrial tissue to grow.

Another drug category that offers promise for the treatment of endometriosis is oral aromatase inhibitor, currently approved for treatment of breast cancer, another estrogen-dependent disease. This drug suppresses aromatase, an enzyme found in endometrial tissue that allows it to implant on reproductive and nearby organs. This tissue then makes its own estrogen. Researchers are currently conducting a nationwide study on the use of aromatase inhibitors as a treatment for recurrent, progressive endometriosis.

Another drug, terbutaline, currently used to prevent premature labor, is also being tested. It relaxes the uterus and prevents abnormal contractions. The drug goes directly to the uterus, and studies show it may be useful for menstrual pain related to endometriosis.

A wide variety of additional medical therapies are being evaluated in noncontrolled clinical trials. One promising drug is the GnRH antagonist, which differs from GnRH agonists because it inhibits the action of gonadotropin-releasing hormones on the pituitary gland, thereby reducing the production of estrogen. The FASTER Study (First Abarelix-Depot Study for Treating Endometriosis Pain Rapidly) is studying women at approximately 50 clinical trial sites throughout the United States to determine if a drug in this category is safe and capable of relieving pain associated with endometriosis faster and with fewer side effects than current therapy.

If you wish to learn more about drug research or take part in a clinical study, contact the Endometriosis Research Center, the Endometriosis Association, pharmaceutical companies, or search the Internet. (See the appendix for contact and resource information.)

Surgery

While medication is often able to control small endometrial growths and mild discomfort, moderate or severe endometriosis, accompanied by extreme pain, may not respond to medication. So, surgery may be recommended. Depending on the severity of growths, a surgeon has several options.

Surgery is used to remove adhesions, so organs are no longer "stuck" together. During surgery, endometrial lesions can be excised (removed entirely) or ablated (destroyed by using a laser, light beam, or other tools). Ablation, generally done with a laser, burns off the surface of the lesion. While this is the most common technique used, it often leaves disease behind. Excision totally removes the lesion or implant, and it can then be sent for pathology examination. Ablation destroys the entire tissue, leaving no sample for pathology.

For superficial implants, ablation may be sufficient. For other implants, however, most experts agree that wide local excision is necessary. Failure to excise deep-seeded implants may cause rapid recurrence of symptoms following surgery or hormone therapy. A skilled surgeon will remove all suspected endometrial growths, not just the black "powder-burn" lesions normally considered characteristic of the condition.

Surgery can range from less to more invasive procedures. The most common procedure, laparoscopy, uses a laparoscope or microlaparoscope to remove endometriosis. Laparotomy, a more invasive procedure, involves a full abdominal incision and requires hospitalization. The most radical surgery is a total abdominal hysterectomy which removes endometriosis, the reproductive organs, and the ovaries.

Let's discuss some of the more common surgical procedures in more detail.

Laparoscopy. Of the surgical options available, laparoscopic surgery is the least invasive, and most conservative; it is usually performed on an outpatient basis. In this procedure, a lighted tube is inserted through a tiny incision in or near the belly button. This allows the surgeon to see inside the abdominal cavity. (This is the same laparoscopic procedure that is used to diagnose endometriosis. For treatment, though, it may be called *operative laparoscopy.*) Alternatively, a microlaparoscopy may be performed in the doctor's office under local or light sedation. This laparascope is the size of a needle, so no incision or stitches are required. Through the laparoscope, the surgeon can drain fluid, destroy growths, free adhesions, or remove large endometrial growths.

Surgery to remove endometrial growths may not always sufficiently reduce pelvic pain. In some more extreme cases, pain is alleviated by blocking the transmission of pain messages from the affected area, primarily the uterus and fallopian tubes. During a laparoscopy, a procedure called a neurectomy may be done with either a laser or electrocautery. A neurectomy in this case is the cutting of nerve fibers that send pain messages from the pelvic area to the brain. Either a presacral or a uterosacral neurectomy or both can be done, depending on where endometrial lesions are located. When a presacral neurectomy is done, the physician strips the nerves in the presacral ligaments (the bands that hold reproductive organs in place and secure them to the spinal column). In a uterosacral neurectomy, the physician cuts the same nerves as in the presacral neurectomy but cuts them closer to the uterus (the uterosacral ligaments).

Laparotomy. The lengthier laparotomy procedure requires a full incision and hospitalization. It is used when there are large implants that cannot be reached with the laparoscope, when pelvic organs such as the bowel are involved, or to remove smaller lesions if a surgeon is not familiar with videolaparoscopy. The incision is usually made along the bikini line.

During a laparotomy, the surgeon can do a number of procedures. These range from removing cysts, lesions, or reproductive organs to destroying adhesions, resecting bowel, or performing a neurectomy.

Hysterectomy. There are different types of hysterectomies, depending on which, if not all, of the reproductive organs are removed. For example, complete removal of the uterus and ovaries is called *radical hysterectomy.* Removing both ovaries is the only way to completely stop production of the estrogen and progesterone. This procedure is called an oophorectomy. It is

believed that removing the hormone-producing body parts will prevent further stimulation of endometriosis and the disease will become inactive. This
"worst case scenario" is usually considered only when all other treatments
have failed. However, even this surgical procedure is not foolproof. As we already mentioned, research has indicated that endometriosis can recur even
after hysterectomy. In one study, 33% of women who had a total hysterectomy
reported that they were not symptom-free after surgery, and 44% of those taking estrogen replacement therapy experienced a return of symptoms.

After removal of both ovaries, estrogen replacement is usually recommended. However, in cases when a woman has a hysterectomy and the surgeon inadvertently leaves behind traces of endometriosis on the cul-de-sac,
the bowel, the bladder, or somewhere else, the endometriosis can return, and
then it may be advisable to stop taking estrogen.

Some doctors may recommend removal of the uterus without removal of
the ovaries. In other cases, surgeons may only remove one ovary because they
don't want to cause early menopause and/or the woman may still be interested
in becoming pregnant. For younger women, surgically induced menopause is
obviously a radical option, especially since hormone replacement (estrogen)
is usually recommended. This can start the whole vicious process all over
again.

Other Surgeries. Like endometrial growths, adhesions cause intense
pain, impair fertility, result in bowel obstructions and bladder problems, and
may require surgical removal. Procedures such as a bowel resection (cutting
a portion of the bowel to remove endometriosis or an intestinal blockage) may
be necessary. Surgery may also be indicated if endometriosis invades portions
of the urinary tract such as the ureter or the bladder. A hysteroscopy, whereby
a scope is inserted into the uterus through the vagina, is another procedure
used to help diagnose problems in the uterus and to pinpoint the cause of
pelvic pain.

Newer Types of Surgery. Newer types of surgery are under investigation. The goal is to improve surgical outcome, while using a less invasive
procedure. For example, surgeons are attempting to use laparoscopy more often to reduce the need for full abdominal surgery. In addition, microsurgical
procedures are being used to treat more delicate structures, free sensitive ad-

hesions, deal with thick scar tissue, or eliminate tiny growths. These techniques require more advanced surgical expertise.

A relatively new procedure called *pain mapping* may help doctors definitively diagnose endometriosis. Unlike the case of traditional laparoscopy, patients are not given general anesthesia but a mild sedative and local anesthetic so they can maintain some consciousness. A microscope is used and the doctor touches the woman's abdominal organs to locate the pain. A recent study showed that this procedure can be helpful for women who suffer chronic pelvic pain that is not relieved with conventional therapies such as nonsteroidal anti-inflammatory drugs (NSAIDs), birth control pills, and antibiotics.

Problems with Surgery. Surgery always has its risks. Although efficient surgical treatment can often provide symptom relief for many years, removing all endometrial growths is often difficult, if not impossible. Microscopic lesions may be left behind. Lesions often return, leading to renewed pain, reduced organ function, and fertility problems. In addition, surgery itself may produce new scar tissue and adhesions. These may all result in pain and require additional surgery at a later date. (See the appendix for lists of things to be aware of to help with your surgical experience.)

THE NONMEDICAL COMPONENTS OF TREATMENT

In addition to the medical treatments we've discussed, there are a number of other ways you can cope with endometriosis. Stress management, proper nutrition, exercise, and various coping strategies can all help improve both your physical and your emotional well-being.

Stress Management

Stress management is an important part of your treatment program for coping with endometriosis. It includes a number of different strategies to deal with both physiological and psychological stress. An important goal in stress management is to improve your feeling of being in control, in terms of your treatment decisions, your emotions, and your behavior, and to reduce pain-exacerbating tension. (See chapter 9 for more information on stress and its management.)

Diet

Proper diet is an important part of a comprehensive treatment program for endometriosis. It is necessary to nourish your body and maintain as much strength and vitality as you can. Good nutrition is a powerful way to optimize health. Nutrition plays an important role in helping you overcome some of the debilitating effects of this disease. (See chapter 15 for more information on diet.)

Exercise

Exercise is another component essential to improving your emotional and physical well-being. Exercise can make you feel better physically, as well as reduce stress and enhance self-esteem. It can also be very helpful in improving the way your body works and the way you perceive your health. Of course, all exercise should be performed only with the approval of your physician or other healthcare professional. (See chapter 16 for more information on exercise.)

Psychological Improvement

Your treatment plan would not be complete without ways to help you successfully cope with the ups and downs of your condition and maintain a positive mental attitude. There are many practical things that can be done to achieve these goals, and we talk about a number of them in more detail throughout the rest of the book.

COMPLEMENTARY/ALTERNATIVE STRATEGIES

Many women are interested in learning more about alternative medicine, also called *complementary* treatments, *nonconventional* therapies, and, by critics, *unorthodox* approaches. Why? Women with endometriosis want to find the best possible ways of coping with this disease. They may want to use alternative therapies to strengthen their bodies and control side effects while undergoing conventional treatment. Or they may prefer a gentler, noninvasive approach—hopefully with fewer side effects. In short, most women with endometriosis want to do everything possible to help themselves, and alternative therapies can be an important component of a comprehensive treatment plan.

You can learn about alternative therapies from a number of sources. By visiting libraries and bookstores, contacting health organizations, and exploring on-line Websites that focus on endometriosis, you should be able to obtain up-to-date information.

Similarities of Alternative Treatments

Even though there are a number of different types of alternative treatments, they do have common themes. Many, for example, are based on the belief that a truly healthy body is much less vulnerable to the ravages of a disease, such as endometriosis. All alternative methods are designed to create (or re-create) the healthiest body possible by reducing or eliminating the vulnerability that allows the disease to develop. The hope is that improved overall health will enhance the body's healing process to eliminate or reduce endometriosis.

Alternative treatments normally use a holistic approach. That is, their goal is to treat the whole body rather than just the area seemingly affected by the endometriosis. Most are based on the idea that although endometriosis may be found in one particular area, the entire body system is involved, so the system must be treated as a whole. Many alternative treatments also work at a number of different levels, including physical, mental, spiritual and emotional.

Types of Alternative Treatments

There are many appropriate alternative treatments that may alleviate the symptoms of endometriosis. For example, some women have found relief with traditional Chinese medicine, acupuncture and acupressure, massage therapy, and herbal remedies. (Additional alternative methods such as biofeedback and imagery are covered in chapter 12.)

Traditional Chinese Medicine (TCM). In this alternative, a natural medical system developed centuries ago, endometriosis is seen as an imbalance of yin and yang, the female and male life forces that run throughout the entire body. It also considers the disease to be a condition of stagnant *energy (chi)* and blood.

Traditional Chinese medicine and Western medicine can work very well together to help some women who suffer from endometriosis. For example, TCM can be used after surgery to facilitate the recovery process, and treatments do not interfere with most modern pharmaceuticals. Traditional Chinese medicine encompasses the treatment methods of acupuncture, Chinese herbs, dietary change, and massage techniques in different combinations. Traditional Chinese herbs come in their raw form, such as sliced root or bark, and are boiled for a period of time. They may be consumed as tea or are available in pill, capsule, or powdered forms. They should be prescribed by and obtained from a licensed practitioner.

Acupuncture/Acupressure. Acupuncture or acupressure are examples of traditional Chinese medicine. Acupuncture is administered using very fine needles inserted into specific body points. Acupressure is a form of massage that applies finger pressure on acupuncture points. Practitioners often use a combination of these methods. Both are used to stimulate or sedate the body's flow of vital energy (chi) along channels or meridians. This helps disperse and dissolve any kind of blockages that may be in those meridians. With endometriosis, the belief is that anything that improves immune system functioning and increases the flow of energy in the body is likely to help.

Herbal Remedies. The medicinal benefits of herbs have been known for centuries. Working with herbs, making herbal preparations and using them for health and healing, can be very therapeutic. Herbs are effective when used over an extended period of time to strengthen the immune system. Herbs are also powerful *adaptogens*, which means that they help the body to adapt to the ever-changing environment and the stresses of life. For women with endometriosis, they are excellent complementary choices. They provide necessary support for the body while it is undergoing more radical forms of treatment that may sap its life energy.

Herbs can be used in many ways—as compresses, teas, essential oils for massage, extracts for oral ingestion, powders, syrups, or salves. There are numerous herbs that are recommended for women who suffer from endometriosis, including alfalfa, dong quai, and red raspberry leaf. They are best used in combination with conventional medical or surgical treatments to reduce estrogen levels and regulate hormonal production in the body (more about these herbs in chapter 15).

Massage Therapy. Massage may be the most ancient and natural pain reliever of all. Massage offers many physical benefits, such as decreasing muscle tension and stiffness, lowering blood pressure, stimulating circulation, and relieving pain. Therapeutic massage is deep and relaxing and gives our bodies a chance to rest and sleep (a time for repair and healing). Some people believe that healing energy is locked in the muscles and that a massage will release energy blockages and help eliminate chronic pain. (See chapter 12 for more information about massage.)

Choosing a Treatment That's Right for You

Your first step for treating endometriosis to learn about medical and surgical alternatives. It's important to fully understand what is available, why your doctor recommends it, and both the benefits and possible side effects. Even if you feel you would prefer an alternative treatment, you owe it to yourself to explore all your options. How you choose to treat endometriosis depends on your individual needs. Perhaps you may try natural therapies before surgery or using hormonal therapy.

In learning about medical or surgical treatments, you'll probably find your doctor or other healthcare professional to be a valuable resource. Don't hesitate to ask about alternative treatments as well; they may know patients or other professionals who have experience with less conventional treatments. If your doctors can't help you evaluate alternative therapies, contact educational organizations, patient referral services, support groups, or Internet Websites for information. As with any healthcare professional, it is important to find a practitioner with whom you feel safe and comfortable.

If you're very interested in alternative therapies and your doctor seems skeptical (or even discouraging), you may wish to locate a more sympathetic doctor or other healthcare professional. If you have difficulty finding a doctor who is willing to support you in your use of alternative therapies, you will have to assume even greater responsibility for your own well-being and conduct your own research.

When screening alternative practitioners and clinics, determine success rates by asking how many cases of endometriosis they see every year. Keep in mind that an effective alternative therapy for one woman's disease won't necessarily be effective for yours. Request supportive studies, documented cases, and patients' testimonials. View all information with a healthy dose of skepticism, and inquire about long-term improvement, short-term improvement, or reduced pain. Also ask if the therapy is being used instead of, or in addition to, conventional treatment. Widely respected healthcare practitioners are increasingly combining the best aspects of conventional medicine with supportive alternative treatments.

Finally, consider whether a therapy fits your own individual lifestyle, personality, and belief system. Some, for instance, may require a degree of practical, emotional, or financial commitment that you are unwilling or unable to make. Others may require more time than you have available, require too much travel, or be too expensive.

What Is Your Role in Treatment?

As you follow your treatment regime, do your best to follow it completely and accurately and be an active participant. Be alert to your progress, and keep an open mind. Feel free to look into other options if the treatment you're using isn't improving things or seems to be working against you.

Physicians and other healthcare professionals can provide medical information, medication, surgery, and expertise. Family and friends can offer emotional support, caring, and guidance. But you are the only one who can make the many important decisions necessary to organize your life as well as possible. These decisions may be small, but they are often critical in determining the effects endometriosis has on you and your family. Obviously, you play a key role. But that's not enough. A whole package approach is essential, where you help yourself in as many ways as possible, both medically and psychologically. The rest of this book will discuss dozens of ways you can help yourself to improve your life with, or despite, endometriosis.

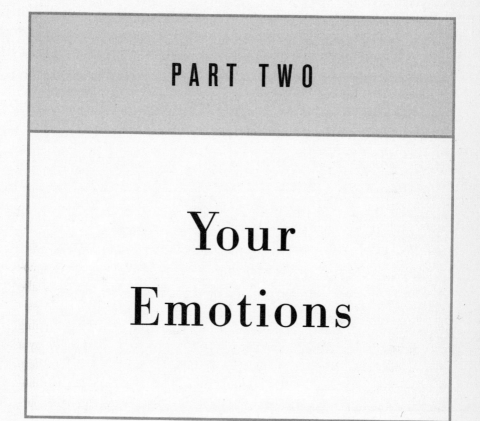

PART TWO

Your
Emotions

CHAPTER THREE

Coping with Your Emotions—an Introduction

How do you feel about having endometriosis? The diagnosis can have a tremendous emotional impact on you, your family, your friends, and everyone around you.

Every person's emotional responses to endometriosis are different. Even your own reactions to this condition will vary from time to time. The more severe your reactions, the more they will interfere with your ability to cope. Your emotions can be like a roller coaster. In other words, you may feel fine sometimes and very upset and panicked at other times. As a matter of fact, emotional ups and downs are very common. And one of the most important aspects of coping with endometriosis is the ability to control your emotions.

Your emotional responses to endometriosis may start even before treatment. Of course, your reactions will depend partly on how suddenly you learned about your disease. For example, if you only recently experienced pain without any advanced warning symptoms and then were diagnosed with endometriosis, you might have a harder time adjusting than if you had been in pain for awhile and suspected a problem. Other factors, such as age and your personal goals, will also help shape your response.

The Factors Shaping Your Emotional Reactions

A number of factors may play a role in determining how you react to endometriosis. Keep in mind, though, that because there are so many factors, no one can predict just how a person will react at any given time. How did you handle problems before your disease was diagnosed? What was your general coping style? Were you calm or nervous? Were you persistent, or did you give up easily? How did you handle pain? The way you've handled life's problems in general will suggest how well you will cope with endometriosis and help you to identify which areas you'll want to improve.

Your age will also have a bearing on how you respond emotionally. Your general physical health prior to the onset of endometriosis, too, will play a role in determining your coping ability. What about your relationships? In many cases, your emotional reactions may reflect the responses of significant others in your life. For example, if family members or friends are anxious or non-supportive, this may have an impact on the way you feel.

Emotional Problems

Have you been experiencing intense anger because you have this disease? Are you angry that your life will change or that it has been in turmoil because of endometriosis? Are you worried that you'll always be in pain? Are you afraid of the treatment you may need—and the possibility of recurrence? Are you worried that you will not be able to afford treatment? Are you afraid of not being able to cope? Do you become depressed when you compare your present life with the way things used to be or with the way it is for other women?

Virtually everyone who is diagnosed with endometriosis becomes anxious, frightened, and depressed. Feeling this way doesn't mean that you are weak. Rather, it means that you are normal! But other than these specific emotional responses, what else might you be experiencing?

You may become disoriented, as if the things around you are unreal. One of the most frightening feelings is that you're not in control, especially if you don't know why you are disoriented. Experiencing severe pain can be very frightening. You may wonder sometimes "What is happening to my body? Am I going to die?" It can be reassuring to understand that this happens to many women with endometriosis from time to time. And it can go away.

How about mood swings? Do you ever experience these? Many women with endometriosis do. But if you stop and think about it, everyone experiences mood swings from time to time—you probably did even before your diagnosis. Certain treatments or medications may increase the range or frequency of these swings. Be sure to let your physician know what you are experiencing and feeling.

The Process of Adjusting

You and your family will probably experience a number of major emotional reactions as you adjust to endometriosis. Let's take a brief look at some emotions and other feelings you may be experiencing during your adjustment period.

SHOCK AND DISBELIEF

Being diagnosed with endometriosis may be shocking. And as the intensity of the shock wears off, it is quickly replaced by feelings of disbelief. It's hard to believe that . . . you've got a *disease!* This disbelief, though, is actually a calmer sensation than the initial shock and subsequent emotions. It gives you a chance to adjust to what you have heard—in your own way, at your own pace.

Give yourself time. Get a second medical opinion if that would make you feel more secure (more about second opinions in chapter 21). Don't feel that you have to absorb it or, more important, accept it all at once.

DENIAL

It may be very difficult for you to accept the fact that you have endometriosis. So instead of acceptance, you may experience denial. And denial can lead to delays in necessary medical treatment.

Believe it or not, there are times when denial can be positive. How? It can keep you from dwelling on problems. In other words, if there's nothing you can do to improve a situation, why keep thinking about it? Remember that although denial does distort reality, there may be times when distortion is necessary. So denial can be helpful as you get used to dealing with the diagnosis. It may enable you to pursue your normal routine while you're getting used to these unpleasant circumstances. But appropriate denial can become inappropriate if it keeps you from doing what is necessary to help yourself.

Family members may also be in denial. But when they allow denial to continue, they may be unknowingly contributing to your inappropriate way of dealing with the problem.

UNCERTAINTY

There is always uncertainty in our lives. Now you're faced with a new uncertainty—regarding endometriosis treatment, outcome, symptoms, your ability to pursue your work goals, start a family, and so on.

Uncertainty exists regardless of treatment outcome. Even if there is success, what about future outcome, recurrences, and problems? And treatment may work for one problem but not another. Just remember that you are able to move in only one direction at a time. Focus on the certainties in your life. Follow your normal routine if you can. Don't play the role of a sick person. Get on with your life.

DAMAGED SELF-ESTEEM

One of the most important elements of our individual personalities is our self-esteem. The way you feel about yourself is critical and helps you get through daily challenges. Unfortunately, a diagnosis of endometriosis may have a damaging effect on self-esteem.

Do you feel less confident since your diagnosis? Perhaps you notice you're behaving differently or you simply don't feel like your old self.

Many women experience a loss of independence with diagnosis—a sense that they are no longer in control—and this can have a negative impact on self-esteem. For example, you may feel there is little you can do to alleviate pain. The sudden onslaught of medical visits, surgery, medication, treatments, waiting to hear about "the next step"—all these changes might make you feel more dependent. If you allow these feelings to take control, your self-esteem will certainly suffer.

What can you do? Instead of being upset by the things you can't do or the ways in which you are dependent on others, focus on the things you still *can* do! Try to maintain as normal a routine as possible. Take control. Get involved in support groups. Speak to others to find out how they handle these very important issues. If necessary, seek counseling for professional advice.

CHANGING BODY IMAGE

Sometimes women experience negative changes in body image with a diagnosis of endometriosis. Even if no one (other than your doctor!) can see what's going on inside your body, you may feel a change, and this, too, can have a very profound effect on your self-esteem.

What can you do to improve your body image? Remind yourself that any changes have taken place inside of you and you control how they affect you. Most changes due to endometriosis are *internal,* and won't be noticeable to others. The most significant step you can take may be to work on your attitude. Remind yourself of who you are and who you've always been. Feel good about the things that are truly important and minimize the rest.

SELF-BLAME

Do you feel as though you "set yourself up" for endometriosis? Do you worry that you're being punished for something you did—that this disease is the result of some wrongdoing? What's the point of thinking this way? Does it really help you? It isn't true, so why let these thoughts overwhelm you?

There's no question that there is a connection between mind and body. The way you feel can certainly contribute to the way your health either thrives or suffers. Before you spend valuable energy blaming yourself for this turn of events, doesn't it make more sense to focus on ways you can build up your body, correct any problems, and move on? One of the best ways you can do this is to improve the way you deal with your emotions. First of all, you'll want to recognize and remove any self-blame. While it is important to be compassionate toward others, you must also be compassionate toward yourself! Try to focus on what you can do to improve yourself, both physically and emotionally.

NEGATIVE THOUGHTS

It is as important to push away negative thoughts as to eliminate self-blame. The less room there is in your mental attitude for negativity, the more room will open for positive feelings. This will provide you with an important foundation in your efforts to cope with your illness.

Everyone has negative thoughts that lead to the growth and intensity of negative emotions. However, there is no law that says you have to let these thoughts continue! Don't allow them to remain in your head and overwhelm you! Keep challenging these thoughts. Work to turn them around and make them more rational, realistic, and positive. In this way, you'll continue to focus on the positive feelings that are such an essential part of successfully living with endometriosis.

It is a waste of valuable energy to be angry, guilt-ridden, self-blaming, or self-critical. It's now time to harness the energy that goes into these negative emotions by turning it into positive thoughts that can build your strength.

Managing Emotional Reactions

Because emotions play such an important role in your life with endometriosis, you'll certainly want to do the best possible job you can of controlling them. The following actions will help you do just that.

GATHER INFORMATION

Keep up-to-date on the latest information on endometriosis and treatment options. Here's a key point: people are usually more afraid of what they don't know than what they do know. The more you know, the better you will be able to help yourself, both in dealing with others and in controlling your own emotional state. Become your own expert on all possible treatment options—both the traditional medical and surgical techniques and the alternative therapies. Use your knowledge to find the most informed healthcare professionals whom you trust, and share updated information with them whenever you think it is appropriate.

Make sure to obtain current, accurate information. The Endometriosis Association and the Endometriosis Research Center are excellent resources, because their information is consistently updated. Attend support groups and informational meetings because, in all likelihood, other attendees will have varying degrees of access to current, helpful information. If you surf the Web, make sure that the information you review is reputable, either written by knowledgeable professionals or posted by legitimate organizations.

JOIN A SUPPORT GROUP

Self-help or support groups, especially those run by professional leaders or facilitators, can be incredibly helpful and are one of the best sources of support and information for women with endometriosis. In fact, research has suggested that support group participants tend to cope better with their disease, and even live longer! Groups provide a forum for the exchange of feelings and ideas. Perhaps most important, these groups will show you that you're not alone, which makes it easier to live with a difficult problem. It's helpful to meet new people, other than family and friends, who know what you're going through because they've gone through it themselves.

Members of support groups all have a common goal: to learn how to live as best they can and to remain as active as possible. You'll see how others handle problems, some of which may be the same as, or at least similar to, your own. This can be a tremendous source of support.

Do you ever feel shunned or ignored by others, or do you fear feeling this way? Are your social relationships dwindling? These groups can give you a feeling of belonging. They may even help educate your family and others, like your employer.

Support groups are great places to share your feelings and gain valuable information and coping strategies in a constructive, therapeutically beneficial way. Remember that groups are not designed to give false hope. They are meant to enable you to express and share real feelings, to learn real strategies, and to derive hope from individuals living in similar circumstances.

In groups, any topics you'd like to talk about can be discussed. You may begin to share feelings more openly when you hear others talking about subjects you were previously reluctant to address yourself. As a result, a feeling of closeness—almost a family feeling—will develop.

Often, members of groups dealing with chronic medical conditions discuss feelings of hostility toward the medical profession. A woman experiencing these feelings may have a hard time communicating with and trusting her physicians. (Chapter 21 contains more information on coping with physicians.) If you should choose to join a support group, it is possible to come away with negative feelings or to realize that the group is not objective. If this happens, report it to the contact organization and ask for additional support resources.

Don't feel that you *must* be in a group. If you're really uncomfortable with the idea or you don't think it's necessary because you're involved in other support activities, that's okay. Just make sure that you're honest with yourself. Don't feel that you have to share your emotional reactions with others. But do realize that these emotions need to be recognized and worked through. That's the only way to make progress.

The list of resource groups in the appendix will help you find a group that specifically focuses on endometriosis. In fact, there are over three hundred local support groups in the United States. The Endometriosis Association and the Endometriosis Research Center provide education, research, and support on both the local and international level. It may also be worthwhile to contact sources such as local hospitals, your physician or other healthcare providers, the state medical society, local schools of psychology or social work, religious organizations, libraries, and the Internet. Or you can always start a group of your own! The Endometriosis Research Center or the Endometriosis Association will be glad to help you start a group in your area, if one does not already exist, or refer you to an existing one.

GET THE BEST MEDICAL CARE POSSIBLE

Make sure you're getting the best possible medical care. If you haven't already done so, you'll want to establish a good working relationship with a physician. Start by finding a doctor who not only has expertise in treating endometriosis and has kept abreast of the latest research but is also understanding, available, and sympathetic to your emotional needs. You can contact the Endometriosis Research Center, or the Endometriosis Association, two organizations that specialize in the treatment of endometriosis. (See chapter 21 for tips on creating a good relationship with your physician.)

LEARN ABOUT MEDICATIONS THAT CAN HELP YOU COPE

There are times when emotions may get too intense, and you may want to consider medications that can help you cope. A number of medications can be effective in dealing with depression, anxiety, anger, and many other emotional reactions to endometriosis or its symptoms. Antianxiety medication, mood el-evators, and antidepressants can be helpful. (More about this in chapter 13.) If you feel that you might benefit from medication, be sure to discuss the pos-sibility with your doctor.

EXPLORE PROFESSIONAL COUNSELING

Professional counseling can help whenever some aspect of your life becomes overwhelming, your emotional problems become severe, or you want to pre-vent problems from getting worse. Certainly, any period of change can be made easier with the help of a support professional such as a psychologist, psychiatrist, social worker, psychiatric nurse, or pastoral counselor or another professional with the necessary credentials, compassion, and expertise.

When speaking to your counselor, it may be one of the few times when you can be totally honest and at the same time get feedback that can help you bet-ter deal with your feelings. Yes, it can be helpful to talk to family and friends and to other people in your situation. But none of these people can provide you with the kind of frank intervention available from a therapist who is fa-miliar with the feelings that endometriosis can create.

If you don't know of an appropriate professional, you can get a referral from any of the physicians who are treating you, from your local support group, or from a local hospital or professional organization.

Of course, not everyone needs professional help. You may do very well on your own.

USE EFFECTIVE COPING STRATEGIES

There are a number of coping strategies you can use to better manage the emotions that may be troubling you. Any of these strategies can help you feel more in control and less depressed.

Make a conscious, constructive agreement with yourself. Tell yourself that you're going to set aside a little time each day to work on strengthening your emotional self and preparing for the next day. During this special time, in-clude activities such as relaxation, imagery, meditation, reading, goal-setting, or positive thinking to improve your attitude. By consciously devoting time to this, you not only will improve your overall emotional state but will also in-crease your feelings of control.

Develop a Positive Mental Attitude

We cannot overstate the importance of a positive mental attitude. Individuals with good mental attitudes can more easily control their emotions. A negative mental attitude may exacerbate any emotional problems you experience. Your primary goal should be to do all you can to change your attitude so that you can improve every other aspect of your life.

Concentrate on the good things. Why waste valuable time and energy focusing on the bad? Always have hope; it is an integral part of the will to live. And research has clearly shown that the will to live plays an important role in the response to treatment for any illness.

The best source of hope comes from within yourself. You can always nurture hope on the basis of what you hear from others. But hope has to start inside of you. This hope will remain strong as long as you're willing to do what you can to sustain yourself and fight for quality of life. Although it may seem like a Herculean task to improve your attitude when you're in severe pain, the goal of developing a positive, optimistic attitude is important.

Books may be very helpful in your efforts to generate a more positive mental outlook. Many offer excellent suggestions. Look into some of these. If you get just one good idea out of a three-hundred-page book, the effort is worthwhile.

Do whatever you can to emphasize the positive. If your attitude is positive, you'll feel better, regardless of what's going on around you. Isn't that worth the effort? Keep up your appearance, and try to be cheerful. Believe it or not, the very act of seeming cheerful often leads to feeling this way. So walk tall and hold your head high. Feel good about who you are.

Laugh a Little

Laughter is one of the most effective coping strategies. Research has shown that chemicals called endorphins—our body's own natural painkillers—are released by the brain whenever we laugh. Endorphins can block pain and give us a feeling of well-being. Haven't you felt better and less tense after having a good laugh? You can enhance the process of getting and staying better by developing your sense of humor and making laughter an important part of your treatment program.

Humor is a pleasurable and effective way to deal with emotions, whether you're listening to someone else's joke, laughing at yourself, or telling your own joke. Although there isn't anything funny about having endometriosis, it helps to look on the bright side and lighten up a bit.

Humor works in three ways. First of all, it reduces anxiety. Laughter is one of the best ways known to release tension. This is important because tension exacerbates pain, while relaxation reduces it.

Second, laughter can distract you from feelings or thoughts that are bothering you. When you're involved in something humorous, you often feel a lot better. Think back, for example, to a time when you were depressed or uncomfortable, and somebody asked if you had heard a certain joke. Initially, you may have been reluctant to hear it. But before long, you were probably totally absorbed in the joke, wondering what the punch line would be! The fact that humor can distract you also means that it can help you see things from a different perspective. So you may be able to look at something more objectively, which can help you handle it more effectively.

Finally, the ability to laugh at yourself is a helpful coping strategy. And it's an important part of maturing. The degree to which this works, however, depends on what you're experiencing. It's just about impossible to laugh at yourself while you're initially going through this crisis. However, as you adjust to your condition, you will better be able to use humor as a coping strategy.

So make laughter-filled experiences a part of your everyday life. Watch funny shows on television. Borrow humorous videotapes. Read amusing books or magazines. Listen to comedy tapes. Read the comics. Any of these things will help you have fun and feel better. Not only can they give you a quick boost by helping you distance yourself from what may be troubling you, but they can also improve your overall mood and physical well-being.

Set Goals for Yourself

Goal-setting can be a very good way of coping with your emotions. What types of goals might you set? A good short-term one might be the purchase of a new book by one of your favorite authors. A long-term goal could involve the planning of a family vacation or activity or, perhaps, a reunion with out-of-town friends. By setting realistic and positive goals and working to achieve them, you'll be giving yourself pleasurable events to anticipate and a reason for getting through every day.

Be Nice to Yourself

Because you've been diagnosed with endometriosis, you may feel that you've given up some control. You may even feel—incorrectly—that you're being punished. It can be very helpful to offset these feelings by emphasizing the fact that nice things can still happen. Often it is important for individuals with chronic medical conditions to be just a little bit more "selfish"—that is, to initiate the kinds of activities or changes that will make them feel better. Of course, this should not be done in a way that is offensive to others, but in a way that states repeatedly, "I am a worthwhile person, and I deserve to have nice things in my life."

What are some of the ways you can be nice to yourself? Consider buying little goodies, taking time to relax, involving yourself in favorite activities, spending more time with the people you enjoy, and so on. You may want to make a list of the things that would be most interesting and pleasurable for you.

Be Nice to Others

Sometimes one of the best ways to boost your own self-esteem is to be nice to other people. The feeling of pleasure you get from helping others can be very gratifying and can improve the way you feel about yourself.

Visiting people in hospitals, nursing homes, and the like is one way to spread sunshine. Performing voluntary services in such organizations as churches, schools, and civic organizations is another possibility.

Helping others will make you feel better about yourself not only because you're performing a kind deed but because you're doing something tangible to better cope with your disease. Helping others with endometriosis can make a big difference in your life. You'll feel more productive. You'll feel like you belong and are an important member of society. Perhaps just as helpful, you'll reduce boredom, possibly make new friends, and channel any excess energy or tension.

Derive Comfort from Faith and Spirituality

People with strong religious faith often derive a tremendous amount of solace from prayer. The religious beliefs of family and friends can also be a source of comfort. However, the degree to which you exercise your religious beliefs is up to you. Don't feel that you have to turn to religion if this does not seem natural to you. On the other hand, if others have religious beliefs, let them derive the comfort and support this provides for them, even if you don't share their intensity.

Make Use of Relaxation Techniques

Tension exacerbates pain; relaxation reduces it. While relaxation procedures alone will not totally control your emotions, they will help you to identify the problems affecting you and allow you to better deal with them. Relaxation procedures can be an essential first step in coping with your emotions.

How can you relax? We're talking about clinical relaxation now—not everyday activities like reading, gardening, listening to music, or sitting in front of the television with a cup of herbal tea. There are several different types of clinical relaxation procedures, including progressive relaxation, meditation, autogenics, deep breathing, and a technique called the Quick Release. All of these techniques are discussed at length in chapter 12, along with imagery, hypnosis, and biofeedback—three techniques that can be used for a number of different purposes, including relaxation.

Remember that if you have difficulty learning to relax on your own, there's nothing wrong with working with a professional who can help you learn these skills.

Pinpoint What's Bothering You

Are you more comfortable now? Good—you're ready to proceed to the next crucial step: in order to deal with tension, you have to determine exactly what is bothering you! Make a list of possibilities. In reviewing your list, you'll see that just about every item can be placed in one of two categories. The first category contains the "modifiables"—the problems or emotions that you can control. The second category includes the "nonmodifiables"—the things you can't control. Why separate them? Because different strategies should be used to deal with each of these two types of problems.

For the first category, you'll want to figure out what techniques you can use to improve the situation. As for the second category, you'll still be planning strategies of a different kind. Where do your emotions exist? In your mind, right? Therefore, your plan for this category is to work on the way you're thinking.

Work on Your Thinking

How can you change your thinking? The technique you choose should depend on the specific emotional reaction that's bothering you. For example, if you're afraid of something and you want to conquer this fear, a procedure called systematic desensitization may be helpful. We'll go into this in chapter 6. Then again, if you're feeling guilty or angry about something, or if something is depressing you, it can be very helpful to learn how to change or "restructure" the way you're thinking. You'll learn more about techniques for this in chapters 5, 7, and 8.

How do you deal with uncertainty? One of the first things to do is to focus on living as a woman who happens to have endometriosis, rather than seeing yourself as a victim. Try to live life fully and enjoy it as much as possible. Concentrate on what you have rather than dwelling on things you don't have. Focus on what you can do each day, not what you can no longer do. Endeavor to live one day at a time, making the most of each day.

Actually, any of the techniques we've discussed can be used to cope with just about any problem. It's simply a question of deciding what works best for you.

What About The Future?

Remember that you are the same person you were before you were diagnosed. The fact that you have endometriosis doesn't mean that anything else about you has changed. Keep this in mind and try to maintain as much control over your life as possible.

Even if you are presently experiencing intense emotional reactions, have faith that these feelings will diminish, either with time or by your doing something to help yourself. On the other hand, anticipate more emotional reactions during times when your symptoms are more pronounced. Even then, you should be able to identify many positive things in your life to help alleviate these feelings. In this way, you can develop a positive mental attitude that should be an integral part of your life.

The purpose of the following seven chapters is to help you to understand different emotions you may be experiencing. You'll discover where these emotions come from and recognize that many other individuals have experienced exactly what you're going through. In addition, a number of strategies will be presented to help you cope with these emotions. Just reading about a method used to control an emotion doesn't guarantee success. You have to keep on practicing. So don't be afraid, depressed, angry, or guilty. Instead, read on!

CHAPTER FOUR

Coping with the Diagnosis

When you first learned you had endometriosis, how did you feel? How did you react when your doctor told you the news? Women may experience a wide range of emotions in response to diagnosis, including anger, fear, and feelings of being out of control. Some cry. Some feel frustration. Others feel numb. Virtually every woman experiences the diagnosis of endometriosis differently. Some take the diagnosis in stride and are actually relieved that it is not "all in their heads"; others are devastated. You may initially feel that it is an obstacle that can never be overcome. Many women diagnosed with endometriosis aren't terribly surprised. They may have expected some medical explanation for the symptoms they're experiencing. Now, at least with a definite diagnosis, treatment can begin in earnest.

Initial Reactions

Let's look in greater detail at some of the more common reactions to diagnosis. Later on in the chapter, we'll look at how you can begin to cope with these emotions.

YOU MIGHT FEEL ANXIOUS!

Immediately after diagnosis, a commonly experienced reaction—and certainly not a pleasant one—is anxiety, sometimes even panic! You may wonder, "Where did it come from? Why do I have it?" You may think, "I'm too young for this." Or you may ask, "What's going to happen to me?" "How will endometriosis affect me?" "What is the treatment—and how will I handle it?" "Will I ever get better?" "Who will take care of me?" "Am I going to die?" You may believe that your life will never be the same again. And family members and loved ones may have the same fears and ask the same questions. They, too, may be anxious as well as helpless, because they don't know what they can do for you. This can certainly make things worse—for them *and* for you.

Let's talk about this reaction. It's normal to be upset and afraid. After all, just the word "endometriosis" can be frightening! You may suddenly be hit with the fact that you are mortal and vulnerable. You'll realize you may have this problem for the rest of your life. Physically, it's not uncommon to feel faint or dizzy or to experience other stress reactions at the time of diagnosis.

Although it may take time to accept the reality of the diagnosis, the process of acceptance began the moment you heard the diagnosis. And acceptance must take place. It is an important step in learning to deal with your condition.

YOU MIGHT BE RELIEVED!

Does everyone feel anxious and afraid when diagnosed? Strangely, no. Some women actually feel relieved to have an affirmation of their symptoms. You might be relieved to rule out the possibility of a tumor or a fatal illness. Sometimes women with endometriosis are mistakenly told they may have ovarian cancer. When the blood test known as CA125 is performed, a false positive result can occur if a woman has moderate or severe endometriosis or ovarian cysts. But laparoscopy often confirms a diagnosis of endometriosis and not cancer.

There are other reasons you might be relieved after your diagnosis. First, you're probably hopeful that treatment will significantly improve the way you've been feeling (and it's good to finally know the cause of your symptoms). Second, family members and friends may have questioned your symptoms, perhaps believing they were all in your head. Unfortunately, some people close to you may still not believe that the problem is physical. They may continue to believe that it is either emotional or stress-related. While you can't force everyone to believe a medical diagnosis, most people's doubts will probably disappear, and strained relationships may improve. Third, and most important, you'll be relieved that *it wasn't all in your head.* After a long period of time, even the most confident person can begin to wonder if there is really something wrong or if the problem is purely emotional.

HOW ABOUT DENIAL?

As we've already discussed, it's not at all unusual to deny that a problem exists. Regardless of the symptoms you've been experiencing, hearing that you have endometriosis may provoke denial. You may believe that your laparoscopy results are wrong. You may feel that the doctor's diagnosis is wrong. You might be willing to deal with the symptoms but not with having a permanent label attached to them.

If you're reading this book, chances are you've already faced the reality of your condition, but if you experience difficulty somewhere along the line, you must seek help. Speak to professionals who know about endometriosis and have them explain it in further detail. Let them tell you about the treatments available for your condition. Or talk to other women with the disease and listen to what they went through when first diagnosed. You will find that many of their experiences parallel your own. You'll also discover that many of them have learned to adjust—just as you'll eventually adjust!

Do you ever ask yourself, "Why can't I go back to the way things used to be?" Do you ever wish you could wake up one morning and find out that this was all just a bad dream? This is very common, but also counterproductive. The more you keep hoping that the situation will go away, the slower your adjustment will be, because you're not really admitting to yourself that things have changed—perhaps permanently. Try to recognize that your condition does exist now, that it affects you, and that it will remain with you. Then aim your efforts in the *right* direction.

HAVE YOU HAD A "DEATH WISH"?

Have you ever wished you could die because your symptoms are so severe and never seem to go away? Some women do. They feel their pain is only going to get worse, interfering more and more with the things they'd like to do, so why bother living? If you've ever felt this way, don't feel guilty. You're not alone. But you should take these feelings seriously and see a mental health professional. Reach out—positive support is out there. Although you may feel like giving up from time to time, these feelings can, *and will,* go away if you work on them. A counselor will help you to focus on all of the positive things you *still* can enjoy in your life, despite the disease.

How Can You Begin to Adjust?

You may have many questions immediately following your diagnosis. Regardless of the way you reacted to your diagnosis, endometriosis is not something that can be ignored. In fact, it's often just as important to be able to conquer your emotions as to address the medical aspects of the disease. It's vital to understand endometriosis, cope with it, and incorporate it into your life—not change your life to fit endometriosis. The most important question is one that only you can answer: "Will I give up living because of endometriosis, or will I continue to live despite my illness?" The following steps should start you on the path to living successfully with endometriosis.

TAKE CHARGE

You must take the reins and begin to help yourself. While you can receive love and support from your family and friends and obtain guidance and expertise from professionals, it's rarely enough. You are the one who is going to have to come to grips with endometriosis. At first, adjusting may be a difficult struggle that requires tremendous effort and emotional turmoil. But there is no other way out. You must face the disease head on.

Even if your initial reaction to the diagnosis of endometriosis is negative, this will pass—usually within a few months. People adjust to the "crisis" of diagnosis and learn that they can cope. However, if you're having an unusually difficult time, don't attempt to simply wait out this period of time until you're OK. You can easily work with your healthcare team or with other women who have endometriosis or get professional help in order to make the transition smoother. Not only will you feel better, but you'll be more productive. Then, later on, if the disease progresses or symptoms worsen you can employ the techniques presented here to help you once again.

INFORMATION, PLEASE!

It's very easy to let your imagination run wild when you hear the word "endometriosis," perhaps for the first time.

Initial anxiety is probably largely the result of not knowing enough about the disease. How serious might it become? How might it affect your family or relationship? If you learn more about the disease, it may seem less frightening. Your physician should be helpful in suggesting ways of getting current information.

After reading current, general, consumer-oriented information, you might want to move on to more technical material. Ask your doctor about anything you don't understand, and certainly ask questions about anything that frightens you. After all, medical writing is not designed to calm the person with endometriosis. It merely states medical facts and statistics. Don't forget this, or you may become unnecessarily alarmed!

It probably wasn't a lifelong goal of yours to become an expert on endometriosis, but think about how much this information may help you. Doctors will respect your questions and opinions. And you'll understand exactly what's going on in your body.

When friends and family first learn of your diagnosis, many will probably send you additional information or try to share stories about others with endometriosis. Although their help is appreciated, make sure that the information you receive is from reputable sources, such as the Endometriosis Association, the Endometriosis Research Center, the United Kingdom Endometriosis Society, or endometriosis groups in other countries. (See the resource list at the end of the book for further details.) And if you find you're receiving too much information, you may want to designate certain members of your family or close friends to be intermediaries for you. Let them go through all the material first, sorting out anything that might be important.

DEVELOP A POSITIVE RELATIONSHIP WITH YOUR DOCTOR

Obviously, you must work with a physician you can trust, one who has had experience working with women with endometriosis. It is definitely beneficial to learn as much as possible about the different treatments for endometriosis. And you can start by asking questions of your physician. Remember that the patient–physician relationship is very important in any chronic illness. If your physician does not seem receptive to your questions, try to impress how important these questions are to you. If no progress is made, then you may have to reconsider this relationship and look for another doctor. (See chapter 21 for more information on working with your physician.)

HELP YOUR FAMILY ADJUST

It is understandably difficult to adjust to the diagnosis of endometriosis and to cope with the many different emotions you are experiencing. This adjustment becomes that much harder when the people close to you also have trouble negotiating the changes the illness brings.

They, too, will go through periods of denial—times when they'll say, "No, everything will be fine" or "I'm sure the problem will clear up by itself." Unfortunately, this won't make things easier for you.

Barbara, an accountant, was 32 years old when she was diagnosed with endometriosis. After a very depressing month, Barbara started to learn how to cope. She was finally able to handle thoughts of lifestyle changes, concerns about pain, and some of the other unpleasant realities associated with her condition. Sound great? Not really. You see, Barbara's husband of 12 years couldn't accept the fact that she had this problem, her two little girls were afraid she was going to die, and her mother had contacted virtually every endometriosis specialist from New York to California! Although Barbara was learning how to cope with her illness, she could not cope with her family. They couldn't handle it, and they were making things very difficult for her.

It's a great idea for family members to seek out help or information. Spouses, children, and others can find out more about endometriosis and learn how others cope with treatment. They can even join support groups or seek counseling. So encourage your family and any willing friends to learn as much as they can and to seek whatever help they need. Their adjustment will help your adjustment.

ADD TO YOUR SUPPORT SYSTEM

Despite mixed emotions from family and friends, their support will generally be of great value to you. This is not a time to be alone. It's the time to reach out—to get support from people you love. Support groups, the Endometriosis Research Center, the Endometriosis Association, and your doctor may be able to help you contact other women with endometriosis in your area so you can talk to them and learn as much as you can.

Summing up

Start thinking positively about your life with endometriosis. Learn as much as you can about your condition. Find support systems and use all the stress management and emotional control techniques you can learn. (Many good ones can be found in this book!) Start saying to yourself, "Endometriosis may be a part of my life, but I'm still alive and I'm going to do whatever I can to help myself adjust and live a long, fulfilling life."

If it's necessary for you to make changes in your lifestyle—even major ones—tell yourself that you will make them, and make them willingly! You're going to lead as complete a life as you can. The more quickly you can adjust your lifestyle to fit your needs, the more rapidly you'll be able to enjoy your life. This may be hard at first, and it will certainly take time. But why not be grateful that you're not helpless and that you can take steps to make the most of your life despite endometriosis!

CHAPTER FIVE

Depression

Lori was feeling very down. A 35-year-old mother of two, married for 12 years, and living in a comfortable home in a good neighborhood, she apparently had everything she wanted. But she certainly hadn't asked for endometriosis! She found herself feeling increasingly upset with the changes she had to make. She was tired of the pain and how it interfered with family life. She felt help-less and hopeless. In short, Lori was suffering from depression.

Depression is a serious problem. Although actual numbers vary, at least five million Americans require professional care for depression each year. Be-cause it is so widespread, depression has been nicknamed the "common cold" of emotional problems.

Just what is depression? Depression is an extremely unpleasant feeling of unhappiness and despair. It can range from a mild problem—feeling discour-aged and downhearted—to a severe disorder—feeling utterly hopeless, worthless, and unwilling to go on living. You may believe that there is no rea-son to remain a part of the world. You may be afraid of being a burden to your family and think that everybody would be better off without you. Or you may just feel useless.

Depression can be painful. Imagine how it must hurt to feel (or say), "I wish I were never born. What good am I? I'm not helping anybody around me, and I'm not helping myself." It may seem as if the whole world is against you. Life may seem unfair—a constant struggle in which you never win. And that hurts.

What Are the Symptoms of Depression?

There are a number of possible symptoms of depression. If you notice that you're feeling excessive amounts of sadness, despair, discouragement, or melancholy; if you're unable to eat; if you're sleeping either too much or too little; if you feel totally withdrawn from social activities; if you find yourself crying often, and that's not typical behavior for you; if you're brooding about the past and feeling hopeless—any of these feelings may indicate depression. There are other symptoms. If you're experiencing excessive amounts of irritability or anger; if your fears seem to be extreme; if you feel inadequate and worthless; if you are unable to concentrate on virtually anything in your life, whether it be work, family, or other interests; if you seem to have little or no interest in activities that previously gave you pleasure; if you have reduced amounts of energy that don't seem to be related to the disease or treatment; if you have little or no interest in sex or intimacy; and if your cognitive style (the way you speak, think, and act) seems to be generally slowing down—these, too, can be symptomatic of depression. The more of these symptoms you experience, the more likely it is that you are depressed and should take some action to help yourself.

How Does Depression Affect You?

Now that you are familiar with some of the many possible symptoms of depression, you should also be aware that its effects are not isolated problems. Depression can affect your physical well-being, take control of your moods, and make it difficult to enjoy—or even carry out—the simplest activity. Let's take a look at some of the ways in which depression can affect you in your day-to-day life.

HOW DEPRESSION AFFECTS YOUR BODY

Some of the more noticeable symptoms of depression are physical in nature, for example, nervous activity, agitation, or wringing of the hands. You may be restless or have difficulty remaining in one place. On the other hand, you may become much less active and remain motionless for abnormally long periods of time, appearing to be almost in a trance, with no apparent desire or energy to do anything.

If you're depressed, most of your physical activities will also slow down—and not just because of physical limitations. You're probably feeling exhausted. This may be surprising, since you're not doing much of anything. But constantly telling yourself that you're no good can be tiring in itself! You really don't want to believe this, but you feel as if you have no choice. And in attempting to escape from these feelings, you may become even more depressed—as well as more physically drained and exhausted.

Depression may also cause you to feel physically sick or experience a change in appetite. Of course, it's wise to remember that any of these symptoms might be related to endometriosis or another physical disorder. So even if the symptoms go away once your depression improves, don't just assume that they're related to the depression. A medical examination may still be a good idea. This way, you'll be sure that there is no organic cause for your depression.

HOW DEPRESSION AFFECTS YOUR MOODS AND OUTLOOK

If you're depressed, you may experience frequent mood swings. For example, you might feel worse in the morning and better in the evening. This nightly improvement may occur because each evening you realize that it's almost time to go to sleep—to escape. But depression may also make sleep difficult, even if you weren't doing much of anything during the day. If you're mildly depressed, you may have difficulty concentrating, and your attention span may be much shorter. When you speak, your conversation may suggest, or even express, feelings of worthlessness and despair.

When you're depressed, it feels as if your mood keeps getting lower. You like yourself very little, if at all. Your thinking is very negative and very different from the way it was when you were feeling good. In fact, it is this negative thinking—not just a particular triggering event—that leads to depression in the first place. (But more on this later in the chapter.)

Naturally, day-to-day activities may suffer as a result of these negative feelings. For example, you might spend the day in your bathrobe simply because you don't feel like dressing. Or you may "go through the motions" of your everyday activities, even though your heart isn't in them. Many people, in fact, simply withdraw from their usual activities during bouts of depression.

HOW DEPRESSION AFFECTS YOUR RELATIONSHIPS WITH OTHERS

Do you now feel less at ease talking to others? Does it seem as if others are having a hard time talking to you, even if they have been close to you for a long time? Because of your depression, you may be less interested in conversation and feel less confident. You may project your negative feelings about yourself onto others and believe that they really don't want to talk to you. And the more depressed you become, the better you get at convincing those around you that you're no good. You may feel that others have no need for you or think that they consider you an uninteresting, boring person.

Marie received a telephone call from her friend Nell. Nell wanted to know how Marie had been feeling. The last time they had gotten together, Marie seemed to be in a lot of pain. Marie responded halfheartedly, imagining that Nell was calling only out of obligation. She then went on to say that she would understand if Nell did not want to call again, because she never seemed to have any good news. How do you think Nell felt? Imagine hearing this repeatedly! Would you be surprised if, eventually, Nell got tired of even trying and simply stopped calling? But in Marie's mind, this would only reinforce her feelings that she really was no good—that she was not worthy of having any friends after all!

What Causes Depression?

A bout of depression frequently starts with one specific thing—an upsetting event or occurrence. Lois had been planning a holiday cruise for over a year. Although she had been in more pain recently, she was still looking forward to the cruise. In the weeks prior to the trip, however, Lois was experiencing so much pain that her doctor advised against her going on the trip. This one disappointment triggered a long depression. Lois felt as if the most important things in her life were being ruined by her endometriosis.

What happens after that first depressing event is a kind of chain reaction. It's almost as if the bottom has dropped out of your world. You may feel that you are less able to control your thinking—although this is not true, as we will show later in this chapter.

Still, a disappointing or upsetting event doesn't *always* lead to depression. So where does it come from, and why does it sometimes take hold? Sometimes we can figure this out, and sometimes we can't. Before we give up, let's discuss some of the possible causes.

WHAT ABOUT THE "NORMAL DOWNS"?

A certain amount of depression is normal in anyone's life. We all experience ups and downs. If we never experienced some of the downs, how could we fully appreciate the ups? However, when depression becomes more than just the "normal downs," it must be addressed.

Of course, certain events—traumatic experiences such as losing a loved one, being diagnosed with a chronic medical problem like endometriosis, anticipating major surgery, or being fired from a job—can lead anyone into a depression. However, this doesn't mean that you should ignore the problem or wait until it goes away. It's necessary to learn how to deal with depression. This is an essential part of coping.

WHAT ABOUT ANGER YOU CAN'T EXPRESS?

What if you get so angry that you feel like you're going to burst—and you don't, or can't, do anything about it, so you decide to "swallow" your anger? It seems strange that a powerful emotion like anger can turn into a withdrawn, helpless feeling like depression. But it can. If you become increasingly angry about something and feel unable to do anything about it, you may turn that anger inward. You may experience so much frustration or hopelessness that you "shut down" in an attempt to keep yourself from experiencing these terrible feelings. This leads to withdrawal, which is one symptom of depression. (For more information on anger, see chapter 7.)

COULD IT BE A CHEMICAL IMBALANCE?

In a small percentage of cases, depression may be caused by biochemical deficiencies—chemical imbalances in our bodies. However, this does not occur very often. Treatment for biochemical deficiencies may involve the administration of drugs in an effort to rebalance body chemistry. But this usually isn't the answer. Regardless of whether your depression is caused by this or, more typically, by your reaction to the people and events around you, you should still try to modify your thinking. Many experts believe that even if the cause of depression is biochemical, by working on the way you handle your day-to-day living, you can have a positive effect on your emotions.

ENDOMETRIOSIS AS A CAUSE

Can endometriosis cause depression? Are you kidding??? The pain and other symptoms of this disease can certainly either create or magnify already existing depression. So it is not surprising that a certain degree of depression can almost be expected if you are living with endometriosis. Depression sometimes even starts before diagnosis, and can reappear periodically. This is totally normal, and is something you'll want to work on to minimize the frequency and length of the "episodes."

One contributor to depression in women with endometriosis is frustration in their need for control. Most people have the need to master at least certain aspects of their life, and endometriosis may make you feel that you've lost control. But even though it may be difficult to admit to yourself that you may not be in control of everything, remind yourself that you can still control certain things. It's much better to focus your energy in this direction.

You may also experience a feeling of helplessness. You may feel weak, uncertain about the future, and powerless to help yourself. This can certainly lead to depression.

What else about endometriosis may depress you? You may become depressed thinking about the future and wondering how endometriosis will affect your life. Worrying about the uncertainties of treatment can be depressing. You may get despondent if you are unable to become pregnant. Problems involving other people may depress you, too. For example, you could feel helpless being able to share what you're experiencing and be depressed that others don't understand. People may expect more from you than you are able or willing to provide. You may be depressed over the possibility of damaged relationships, lost friendships, or family friction. If you're single, you may be heartbroken at the thought that endometriosis will affect possible future relationships—not that there need be any truth to this at all!

Depression may also result from lifestyle changes. What if you are not able to participate in all of the activities you used to love? What if you have to change your work routine, as well as your family routine? What if you experience money problems? Any of these issues can certainly be depressing.

You may be saying to yourself, "If I'm depressed over my endometriosis, how can I expect to conquer it unless my endometriosis is cured?" This kind of thinking will get you nowhere. You don't want your emotional state to depend on your physical state. So if your depression lingers, don't wait. Work on it, and learn how to cope.

What Maintains Depression?

If you're depressed, you may be blaming yourself—or your endometriosis—for everything that is wrong. You may become more and more withdrawn and pull away from the world around you. Why? Do you believe that if your condition is causing all these horrible things, it is better to "escape" and not think about it? Realistically, though escaping won't solve anything. But you may feel that withdrawal is the only way to stop feeling terrible. Unfortunately, this will only keep you depressed. (In fact, it may make you even more depressed.)

Although others may think that you are sullen and withdrawn, you're probably in deep emotional pain. Part of what is making you, and keeping you, depressed is your effort to protect yourself from this emotional pain. You feel that nothing good can possibly happen—that only bad things can happen. So what do you do? You try to block everything out of your mind!

So why do you stay depressed? Why doesn't it just go away? Maybe you don't want to talk to anybody or even consider counseling. So you keep the thoughts and feelings that lead to your depression inside. You may ask, "Is my unwillingness to talk the only reason I'm still depressed? If I start talking more, will that get me out of my depression?" Not necessarily—but it can certainly be helpful to talk out your feelings. It would probably be beneficial if a close friend or family member took the initiative and forced you into some kind of conversation—therapeutic or otherwise—or at least pushed you into doing something constructive.

How Can You Cope with Depression?

Can anything be done to end depression? Of course! First, tell yourself that the main reason you're depressed is that you haven't yet taken the proper steps toward feeling better! These steps can pull you out of your rut and reacquaint you with the more positive, pleasant aspects of living—the aspects you'd like to experience.

Unfortunately, once you've fallen into depression, it takes hard work and a certain amount of persistence to pull yourself out. The result, however, is surely worth the fight. And, of course, the fight will be easier if you know and use specific techniques and activities that will help. Don't be afraid of depression. Rather, expect it and prepare yourself for it. This will help you better deal with depression when it does occur.

The strategies and techniques that work most to deal with depression can also help to prevent it, although not always conpletely. Future episodes of depression may happen. If you anticipate this, when and if depression does recur, you won't completely fall apart. And if this feeling does come back, won't it be good to know that you *can* do something to help yourself?

One of the first things you must do in learning to cope with depression is to accept whatever limitations exist in your life. Admit that you can't control or become involved in *everything*. This doesn't mean that you are powerless, but it does mean that you may have to alter your views about what you can and can't do. Once you accept your limitations, you'll be able to focus your energy in appropriate, constructive directions instead of lamenting what has changed. How can you accept your limitations? Well, let's say that you were previously able to do twenty-five things in your life and now, because of endometriosis, you're unable to do ten of them. Instead of wasting your energy thinking about the things you can no longer do, focus your energy on feeling good about the ones you can do! Remember the Serenity Prayer: "Grant me the serenity to accept the things I cannot change, the courage to change the things I can, and the wisdom to know the difference."

Another strategy to alleviate depression is to exercise choice. Demonstrating that you have the ability to choose certain things in your life will help increase your feeling of control. Sure, certain events may be beyond your influence, but you can still focus your energy on all the things you *can* do.

Regardless of what you must do and what mountains seem to stand in your way, the most you can ask of yourself—the most that anybody can ask—is to take one step at a time. Just keep taking one more step. This will be helpful, especially if you're feeling overwhelmed.

Now that you're ready to fight your depression, consider two major ways of dealing with it: being more physical (in other words, doing something) and working on your thinking. It can be very helpful to make a list of all the things that are depressing you. You may feel there will be at least fifty items! But in actuality, you'll probably start running out of ideas after six or seven. Next, divide this list into two more: first, those things that you can change, and, second, things you can't. Get physical and do something about the items on the first list, and get thoughtful—work on your thinking—regarding the items on the second list.

LET'S GET PHYSICAL

There are two ways of getting physical in order to deal with depression: actively working to accomplish goals and increasing physical activity. Hopefully, as suggested, you've listed all the things that are depressing you, and all the things that can be changed. Now think about ways you can modify or eliminate items. Be realistic but aggressive and plan to reach your goals.

Where does the physical activity enter? Unknowingly, you may be using a lot of energy to keep yourself depressed. You may be working hard to keep that anger inside, even if it appears to others that you're simply withdrawing. If your depression is anger turned within, we can logically assume that by releasing your anger, you'll be able to eliminate your feelings of depression. But what should you do with those feelings? You must find an object toward which you can express your anger. This may be difficult. However, it's important to release the trapped anger so that it doesn't build up and deepen your depression.

Think about the following scenario. You're sitting there, depressed and withdrawn. Somebody makes an innocent remark, and you practically bite that person's head off! What's happening? Whatever was said triggered the release of the internalized anger that was making you depressed. Look out, world!

What can help you release your anger? Many physical activities can, depending, of course, on what you're physically able to do. Try walking, playing golf, tennis, or swimming. Yoga, meditation, or exercise classes are great ways to release anger. Be sure to get your doctor's okay, if necessary, before beginning any exercise program. (For more information on coping with anger, see chapter 7. For more information on exercise, see chapter 16.)

LET'S GET THOUGHTFUL

Although getting physical may help lift your depression—and can also provide a great distraction, which may help you to look at things more objectively—physical activity will not teach you ways of fighting inappropriate thinking. Remember that it's your *thoughts* that have made you depressed. Clearly, restructuring your thinking is a key element in alleviating depression and dealing with any negative emotions.

If you can think yourself into depression, then obviously you can think yourself out of it. How? If you're depressed, you're just talking yourself *down*. All your comments—or at least most of them—are probably put-downs: harsh statements that can make you feel even worse. You want your inner voice to help you, not hurt you. Let's see how you can do that.

Distinguish Fact from Fiction

When you're depressed, you tend to distort reality. Clinical research with depressed patients has proven this. Recognize, therefore, that your thoughts are not necessarily based on what is truly happening but may, instead, be based on your own distorted views. This is called *cognitive distortion.*

Is this bad? You bet your happiness it is! "Cognitive" refers to your thinking. "Distortion" means you're twisting things around and, in general, losing sight of what's real. We all tend to do this from time to time. But when you're depressed, you do it a lot—if not all of the time—and it keeps you depressed. So how do you stop? First, you must become reacquainted with what is really happening. But how can you do that if you keep distorting reality? Right now, you're better off accepting somebody else's perceptions of the situation, because that person is probably a lot more objective and accurate. Depression can be reduced, if not eliminated, once your understanding of reality changes.

Louise kept moaning because none of her friends were calling her. "They don't call as much as they used to. I guess they just don't care." Her sister, Lois, asked her to estimate how often her friends used to call. When Louise compared this with the current number of calls, she realized that it was almost the same. She then recognized that she was probably just more sensitive because she had been feeling depressed! Although she did not feel 100% better, Louise was a bit more cheerful, because she could now see that she hadn't been abandoned.

So make sure you know what's true and what's not. Provide your own assessment of the situation, and be as objective as possible. Then, if necessary, ask other people—people whose opinions you trust—for their evaluation. Work to become more comfortable with any differences in perception and to adjust your thinking so that it more closely resembles the actual circumstances.

Make Molehills out of Mountains

Does this imply that if you're depressed you have no real problem? Is it "all in your head"? No. Everyone has problems. If you feel good, you can handle them; but if you're depressed, you may feel overwhelmed. And when that happens—each and every unpleasant event or symptom you experience, regardless of how trivial or slight it may be, will tend to depress you.

Again, do your best to view each problem objectively—to avoid blowing it out of proportion. Eventually, as your depression lifts, you will be able to deal with all of life's problems, both big and small.

Avoid Self-Fulfilling Prophesies

We've discussed several thoughts that are characteristic of depression—thoughts you may be having right now. While many of these thoughts and feelings may be irrational, ironically, the longer you feel this way, the greater the chance of their becoming self-fulfilling prophecies. In other words, the more you allow yourself to think negatively, the greater the likelihood that your fears will turn into realities. For example, if you begin telling yourself that friends and relatives don't care, this may become a reality, because your negative attitudes may alienate the people close to you. And if you feel less able or less willing to do things, your inactivity is likely to magnify and confirm your feelings of worthlessness, leading to even greater depression and helplessness. Not a pretty picture.

Once you begin feeling depressed, your negative thoughts will soon lead to negative actions. These negative actions will lead to more negative thoughts, which will in turn lead to more negative actions, and so on. It is an ongoing, vicious cycle that will spiral you further downward into deeper depression. Eventually you'll feel trapped in this vicious cycle and believe there's no way to escape.

Are you getting depressed just reading this? In all probability, if you've ever been depressed, you've already said to yourself, "Wow, that sounds just like me!" So if you find that you're starting to believe in your negative thoughts, stop yourself. As we've said already, depression both results from and causes a lot of negative thinking. But once you become aware of these thoughts, you can do something about them. People who remain depressed feel incapable of doing anything about their negative thinking and allow these thoughts to pull them into that vicious cycle mentioned earlier. Try to think positive thoughts, so that if one of your thoughts does turn into a reality, it will at least be a positive one.

Dwell on the Brighter Tomorrows

Although she was physically in good shape, Susan was depressed because she had no idea when she would have pain. She was afraid to participate in activities that she loved, including swimming, staying out late with friends, spending leisurely afternoons in museums, or planning vacations that involved outdoor activities such as skiing and hiking. She allowed her depressing thoughts to overwhelm her, and, as a result, she certainly did not give herself a chance to enjoy life.

If you find yourself thinking along the same lines as Susan, try to modify your thoughts. Start planning fun things for the present and future. Anyone can come up with some enjoyable activities, *regardless* of physical restrictions. But it takes effort. Don't wallow in self-pity, because that will only allow your depression to overwhelm you. Develop some positive plans and translate them into pleasure. Then wave goodbye to your depression!

Of course, if you clearly reflect on your past, you may find that it wasn't much better than the present! In the past, you may have had other physical problems. You may have made some mistakes. Naturally, this may make you even more depressed about the future. However, you can't change the past. What's done is done. Keep telling yourself that. Don't punish yourself for the past. Tell yourself that you're going to work on making the future better. Set up some specific goals, starting with the easy-to-reach ones. You'll be helping yourself just by *thinking* about all the positive things you can do!

Rediscover What's Missing from Your Life

You may have laughed when you read the title of this section. "I *know* what's missing from my life," you might respond. "Healthy insides!" Sure. But another important element that might very well be missing—an element that *can* be regained!—is the feeling of satisfaction, accomplishment, and pride that normally comes from others' praise. You may be missing the attention and interest of other people, and this can cause you to feel worthless. What can you do about it? Think about your positive qualities. (Yes, you do have some!) Think about how you can interact more with people, spark their interest, and obtain more of the satisfaction that makes you feel worthwhile.

Shoot for the Earth, Not the Moon

We all have goals for ourselves. It's normal to become depressed when we don't reach a particular one, especially if we've tried very hard to get there. But sometimes our goals are not realistic.

Try to judge if the goals you've been setting for yourself are realistic. If not, reset them, keeping your abilities and limitations in mind. Once your goals are more realistic, you'll have a much better chance of achieving them and less chance of falling short.

TALK ABOUT IT!

Now you know how to cope with depression through both physical activity and by changing your way of thinking. But there's one more thing you can do—something we've mentioned earlier. You can *talk* about your problems and concerns with others. Often the very act of talking will help lift your depression. If there are family members or friends with whom you feel close and whose opinions you trust, approach them. Air your feelings and listen to their feedback. They may be more objective and better able to come up with constructive solutions.

If your depression is so intense or prolonged that friends and family are unable to help, then by all means consider speaking to a professional. Counseling is becoming increasingly effective for treating depression. So don't deny yourself this invaluable assistance. Why not do everything you can to help yourself feel better?

An Antidepressing Summary

The best way to work on negative thoughts is to prevent them from continuing. Be realistically positive. Deal with reality the way it actually exists. View thoughts from a more factual point of view. Handle them the way somebody else might—who is not depressed and who can be more objective. Try to make your perceptions more accurate, your awareness more realistic, and your thoughts more constructive. Remember: your thoughts lead to your emotions. If your thoughts are negative and critical, your emotions will be the same. But if you can turn your thoughts around to a more positive, constructive point of view, your emotional reactions will most certainly follow. And depression will then be a thing of the past.

CHAPTER SIX

Fears and Anxieties

Don't be *afraid* to read this chapter! It may help you discover what you're *anxious* about!

The two sentences above may help you distinguish between anxiety and fear. What is the difference? Anxiety is a general sense of uneasiness—a vague feeling of discomfort. It is an agitated, uncertain state in which you just don't feel at peace or in control. There is a premonition that something bad may happen, something that requires protecting yourself. You feel very vulnerable. However, you're not exactly sure about the source of your anxiety.

Fear, on the other hand, is usually more specific. It's often directed toward something that can be recognized, whether a person, an object, a situation, or an event. We have fear when we become aware of something dangerous or when we feel threatened. When we are afraid—much as when we're anxious—we feel out of control and less confident. So the feelings of anxiety and fear are basically the same; the main difference is whether the source of the feeling can be identified. Most important, the strategies used to combat fear will also enable you to cope with anxiety. For this reason, from this point on we'll be using the two terms interchangeably.

Fear is so common that we have developed a number of different words to describe it. The important point to remember is that the source of your fear may be either real or imaginary.

Fear and Endometriosis

Unfortunately, women with endometriosis all too commonly experience anxiety and fear. They may be afraid that the pain will never stop. They may worry that endometriosis will affect their social and vocational activities. They may be scared of the treatment, especially if surgery is something that frightens them. Many are fearful of the hormonal drug treatments and their potential side effects. They may worry that they'll never have children, or that if they do, they will pass their poor health on to them. They may even worry about *being* afraid.

Often, the emotions experienced by women living with endometriosis parallel the course of the disease. Feelings are usually the most negative during more painful periods. When you genuinely feel good, emotions may be much more positive. But even during periods of remission, anxiety is common. (For example, you may be afraid of symptoms returning.) And because anxiety can interfere with your ability to deal effectively with any medical problem, it's vital that you learn to cope with this emotion.

The best way to start dealing with your fears is to obtain as much information as you possibly can. By gaining knowledge and understanding, you will equip yourself to fight and conquer your fears. Just as important, both you and your family can implement successful psychological strategies that will help you deal more effectively with your fears, enabling you to better adjust and cope—skills that will help you in many areas of life.

What Are the Symptoms of Fear and Anxiety?

What happens when you become extremely anxious? Your body may react physiologically. You may become short of breath, your heart may beat rapidly, you may feel shaky, and you may think, "I've got to get out of here!" You may attempt to relax but instead stay very tense. You may take a deep breath but find that the breath keeps catching in your throat. You may try to "shake the feeling" but find that you can't. This inability to calm down can be frightening and may increase your anxiety even more. A vicious cycle can quickly develop. Before long, you may feel completely out of control.

Which came first, the anxiety or the symptoms? That's really not important. What's more crucial is doing whatever you can to reduce both. That's what will help you cope with fear—to regain control of your emotions and improve your day-to-day life.

Is Fear Good or Bad?

Believe it or not, fear is usually good! How is this possible? Fear mobilizes you. It tells you to prepare to attack the source of your fear. You react in a way that leads to action. In this regard, fear is similar to stress. It serves a necessary and critical purpose. In a way, it protects you.

Anxiety is bad only when the source of your fear becomes overlooked, ignored, or denied or when the feeling is so excessive that it paralyzes you. In such cases, the threat or danger is allowed to continue, and nothing—or not enough—is done to control it.

What Determines the Intensity of our Reactions?

Fear ranges in intensity from mild to severe. It is impossible to measure just how much fear there is in anyone's life. This varies from person to person and from time to time.

What determines how fearful you get? For one thing, how close is the dreaded object, person, or event? (Wouldn't you be more afraid if you were getting an injection within the next thirty seconds than you would if you were getting one in 30 days?) How vulnerable are you? (Do you truly hate injections, or are you just tired of feeling like a pincushion?) Finally, how successful are you at defending yourself? (Can you calmly accept the needle, or do you scream a lot?) These are just some of the factors that determine how you handle fear.

Jan, age 31, was afraid to go to sleep at night. She was worried that she'd be awakened in the middle of the night by pain, which would remind her of the endometriosis. If Jan had been emotionally stronger, she might still experience some discomfort but would not let this disturb her sleep. Instead, Jan allowed the fear to keep her awake, and as she got less sleep, she became more vulnerable to the very feeling she wanted to avoid!

What Is Panic?

Although this chapter focuses on anxiety and fear, we really can't discuss these emotions without also considering panic. Panic is the most intense form of anxiety—it's what you feel when your anxiety increases beyond the "typical" level. In fact, with panic, the degree of anxiety is so profound that you feel as if you've totally lost control. Research suggests that approximately 5% of the general population suffers from panic disorders.

Panic may strike suddenly and without warning. Occasionally, there may not even appear to be a specific trigger. Or the trigger may be perfectly clear, but you may find yourself unable to prevent the panic attack.

Although there are times when anxiety can be beneficial, panic is usually so intense that there are few, if any, benefits to the experience.

WHAT ARE THE SYMPTOMS OF PANIC ATTACKS?

The most common symptoms of panic attacks are palpitations, increased heart rate and blood flow, pounding heart, chest pain, sweating, dizziness, shortness of breath, imbalance, disorientation, a feeling of suffocation, rubbery legs, flushing, tingling in different parts of the body, faintness, numbness, nausea, shaking, trembling, a lump in the throat, and lightheadedness. Even this sounds frightening! But the list doesn't end here. There are also psychological symptoms, including the feeling of going crazy, fear of dying, fear of losing control, a feeling of impending doom, and an urgent desire to escape.

A number of the physiological symptoms are triggered by sudden bursts of adrenaline, a substance released by the body when you're under stress. This stress response has also been called the "fight or flight" syndrome. (You'll read more about this in chapter 9.)

By the way, it's important to be aware that many of the symptoms of panic attacks may also be symptomatic of mitral valve prolapse (MVP) syndrome, which seems to accompany a structural defect of the mitral valve of the heart. It's important to be aware of this, since MVP is fairly common in women with endometriosis. If you experience any of these symptoms, be sure to discuss this with your physician.

CAN I STOP A PANIC ATTACK?

When you are experiencing a panic attack, it may be very difficult to view the situation rationally and realize that there is nothing to fear—or, at least, that your fears may be out of proportion. Rather, you may be unable to think objectively, and your emotions may take over. The fear then becomes more intense.

The more you feel unable to control panic attacks, the more often they may occur. This happens in part because you're already feeling out of control, so it takes less stress to trigger an attack.

There are times when panic attacks are very short. They may last for only a few minutes and then pass. At other times, though, they may last for up to an hour or more. This can be devastating!

The desire to avoid panic attacks may lead to the onset of phobias. Why? Phobias—irrational fears of a situation or object—actually begin as avoidance behavior. You may start associating the discomfort of panic attacks with whatever situations you were in at the time the attacks began. You'll then try to bypass these situations, becoming phobic in your intense need to avoid the triggers of these attacks.

Fortunately, many of the techniques that help you deal with anxieties and fears will prevent your emotions from escalating into panic. These strategies include pinpointing possible reasons for your fear and panic, using relaxation techniques to prevent or overcome your panic, and restructuring your thinking. If your feelings of panic continue, though, medication or counseling may be necessary. There are also many successful programs that could help you cope with panic attacks.

How Can You Cope with
Anxieties and Fears?

Obviously, the more fears you have, the more difficulty you'll experience in making a successful adjustment to your new situation. Recognizing your fears and learning how to deal with them will help you live more happily and comfortably. How? We were afraid you'd never ask! Let's look at some of the ways you can help yourself better cope with your fears. Later on in the chapter, we'll look at how you can use some of these strategies—and others, as well—to cope with some specific fears that may be troubling you.

PINPOINT THE SOURCE OF YOUR FEARS

The first step in coping with your fears is to use the pinpointing technique discussed in chapter 3. Identify and list exactly what scares you and exactly why you are afraid. Is it not knowing what course your endometriosis is taking and where the pain will next occur? Is it being afraid of anesthesia administered for surgical procedures? Are you afraid that no man will want to marry you with this disease? Then think about what you can do to alleviate your fears. As you begin planning your strategies and gradually putting your plan into operation, you'll begin to feel better.

RELAX!

Because relaxation is the opposite of tension, using relaxation techniques can be very helpful in coping with anxieties and fears. There are many types of relaxation techniques: progressive relaxation, meditation, autogenics, deep breathing, and more. Regardless of what is provoking your fear, learning to relax is an important part of improving emotional well-being. (Detailed information about relaxation techniques can be found in chapter 12.)

DESENSITIZE YOURSELF

One great technique for conquering fear is called *systematic desensitization.* Using this technique, you gradually desensitize yourself—that is, make yourself less vulnerable—to the source of your fear.

Here's how it can work for you. Sit in a comfortable chair and relax. Then create a movie in your mind by imagining whatever it is that makes you afraid. If you get tense, stop imagining it and relax. When you've calmed down, try imagining it again. The more you try to imagine your fear, alternating this "movie" with relaxation techniques, the less your fears will bother you. Try it!

It will give you a great feeling of relaxation and control. There are many books that provide more information on systematic desensitization. Check them out.

LEARN TO COPE WITH ANXIOUS THOUGHTS

Anxiety is a vague, uneasy feeling with an unknown source. So how can you cope with anxiety by following the steps just listed? Surely, if you can't pinpoint the source of your fear, you can't follow these specific steps. So what can you do? Well, a number of things may work. Try the relaxation procedures discussed earlier in this chapter. Work on changing your thinking to make it more positive and productive. Find somebody who will listen to you, talk to you, and help you try to deal with your fears realistically. Even if you can't pinpoint a specific fear, these techniques will greatly help you cope with general anxiety experienced by many women with endometriosis.

LEARN MORE ABOUT ENDOMETRIOSIS

Things that are unknown are often feared. And, unfortunately, there are still a lot of unknowns regarding endometriosis. However, the more people you speak to, the more questions you ask, and the more information you obtain, the fewer "unknowns" there will be. Knowledge is power! The more you know about endometriosis, the possible course your disease will take, treatment options, and the normal symptoms, the easier it will be to eliminate many of your fears, or at least reduce them to the point of being manageable.

Let's Talk About Specifics

When you were first diagnosed, many fearful questions probably came to mind. "What will the future be like? What will become of me?" These are all typical questions of people who are diagnosed with any chronic medical problem, not just endometriosis. As time has gone by, in all probability, some of these questions have been answered and you have started to adjust. But once these initial fears are reduced, others may arise. In other words, you may now focus on the fear of pain, of surgery, and of other possible symptoms, events, and experiences. All of these fears are normal and understandable, and should be expected. But however normal they may be, they can become extremely harmful if you fail to effectively cope.

In the previous pages, we presented some general coping strategies. But you're probably most interested in how these and other strategies can help you better cope with specific fears you're struggling with as a result of your endometriosis.

FEAR OF PAIN

Nobody likes pain. And because pain, unfortunately, is common with endometriosis, you may fear it. Each little twinge of pain may make you afraid—afraid that your condition is not responding to treatment or that additional problems are developing. And even when you're not in pain, you may be anxious about when it will return.

What can you do about this fear? Try to accept the fact that, though you may experience some pain from time to time, medication and other interventions can reduce its intensity as well as its duration. Realize that each pain "cycle" will eventually stop, or at least lessen. The pain won't last forever. (For more suggestions on coping with pain, read chapter 12.) Do you see how you must work on your thinking? If negative thoughts make you more afraid, then positive thoughts . . . !

FEAR OF GOING TO THE DOCTOR

It's not uncommon for women with endometriosis to be fearful of medical visits—both to doctors' offices and the hospital. Instead of hoping that these visits will help them, they may be afraid of what they are going to learn. Or they may have been mistreated, undiagnosed, or dismissed by doctors. In fact, in some cases this fear is so overwhelming that they don't go to the doctor when they should. It's not uncommon for some women to wait weeks or even months before finally making an appointment. Sometimes they may wait years!

As you know, this is definitely unwise. So make and keep your appointments. You're trying to help yourself the best you can, right? So if there's anything that needs medical attention, you'll want to find out so that you can take care of it! That doesn't mean you're going to love all of your doctor's visits, but you do want to make the best of them.

FEAR OF "WHAT NEXT?"

What will happen next? Unfortunately, you can't be sure. Will the endometriosis spread? Will you experience any side effects from your treatment? Will you develop new symptoms?

Everyone wonders what the future will hold. But because of the unpleasantness of what you're experiencing, you may be afraid of the future, rather than merely curious. What can you do? Because you can't foresee what will happen, take life one day at a time. Tell yourself that you'll handle any problems as they occur. Talk with other women who have endometriosis. Keep doing what is necessary to take care of yourself.

FEAR OF TREATMENT

Regardless of which treatment your doctor prescribes, there may be frightening things about it that may upset you.

For instance, you may be concerned about the side effects of medication. Yes, it's true that virtually all medications have side effects (see chapter 13), but you'll want to focus on the benefits. Discuss these concerns with your physicians, ones you know are board certified, well trained, and experienced in the treatment of endometriosis.

You may fear having surgery, worrying about the pain, what it might do to your insides, and that it might not eliminate the problem. You may fear losing your ability to have children. But wouldn't it be better to focus on the anticipated benefits of the surgery—the elimination of endometrial growths from your body?

You must deal with *all* of your fears regarding treatment by asking any questions beforehand. Learn as much as you can. Speak to others who have experienced your prescribed treatment. Make sure you understand the purpose of the treatment, the potential for success, and the fact that there are ways to minimize side effects. By anticipating what may happen, you'll be in better shape to deal with the possible consequences.

FEAR OF RECURRENCE

Even if your endometriosis treatments are successful, you may still have fears. One of the most common fears is that the disease and the symptoms will return. Of course, your doctors will tell you that you have to follow your treatment plan and report any serious problems. This is certainly important. But don't become obsessed with reporting every little twinge. You don't want to become "endometriosis-phobic"! Discuss realistic guidelines with your doctor regarding what you should report and what is not abnormal. And don't let these feelings overwhelm you. Speak to others who have been through it. By all means speak to professionals who are trained to help you deal with these fears. And remember that your goal is to manage whatever occurs, one day at a time.

FEAR OF THE REACTIONS OF OTHERS

Are you afraid that others will shy away from you because you have endometriosis? You may be concerned that you will lose friends. You may even fear being abandoned by your spouse, your fiancé, or other loved ones.

Unfortunately, some people *can* be cold, unfeeling, and insensitive to your problems. But your true friends will accept you under any circumstances. Enjoy them.

Naturally, you should aim to live your life as normally as possible. Remain involved with family and friends. But be realistic. Remember that a change in a social relationship can occur for any reason, not just because of endometriosis! And since you can't change the way some people feel, try not to be too concerned with their reactions. Instead, be more attentive to your own needs and feelings.

Of course, if you think that an important relationship is in jeopardy, you should try to figure out the reason and determine what you can do to improve things. And if you feel that people are shying away from you, try to discuss this with them. Find out what their concerns are. Maybe you'll be able to remedy the situation. Get counseling, if necessary. But remember that you can do only so much. If your efforts don't work, at least you'll know that you did your best.

Finally, if you have been troubled by the reactions of others, you may find it helpful to get involved in a support group. You know that the people in these groups will not shy away from you or abandon you. Why? Because they're going through the same kinds of things that you are! And because of their own experiences, participants may even be able to give you some tips on dealing with family and friends. (For more information on dealing with others, see chapter 19.)

FEAR OF OVERDOING OR UNDERDOING

You may not know how much you should be trying to accomplish. You may be afraid of doing too much but feel guilty about doing too little! How can you conquer this fear? Get advice from experts. You'll need professional guidance to come up with the best "mix" of rest and exercise. And you'll need to know which, if any, activities may be too strenuous for you at certain times.

Of course, even your doctor may not have specific answers for you. You may be told that the answers will become apparent only through trial and error. After all, experience is the best teacher.

So what should you do? Pace yourself. Change your activity level as needed, but try to change it gradually. Then tell yourself that, as with so many other fears, you're doing the best you can. Take pleasure in whatever you may accomplish.

FEAR OF EMPLOYMENT PROBLEMS

Like many women with endometriosis, you may be concerned about the effect your condition will have on your job. You may want or need to work but fear that symptoms will make it too difficult. Your employer may be understanding at first, but you'll probably worry about how long his tolerance will continue. And, of course, your need for money may be greater because of your medical problems! So if you can't work, the pressure can be tremendous.

What can you do? Talk to others who have been in the same situation and see how they have handled it. Speak to experts who can advise you on financial matters. Evaluate your vocational skills and make sure you're equipped to do a job that you can physically handle. Remember, you'll work it out. (See chapter 18 for more about this subject.)

FEAR OF FEAR ITSELF

This section might be called "Fear of Anxiety," "Fear of Panic Attacks," or a number of other things. What they all describe, though, is the response that many people have to anxiety and fear. Because these emotions are so uncomfortable, many people develop a fear of being afraid. This is known as a secondary anxiety reaction. It means that you're not afraid of a specific object, person, or situation as much as you're anxious about being anxious!

What to do? Start by using relaxation techniques. Then tell yourself that you'll approach any situation or feeling as it occurs, rather than worrying about what might or might not happen. Reread the information in this chapter. And, if necessary, work with a supportive professional to help cope with this problem.

FEAR OF NOT COPING

You may feel that you're barely handling your endometriosis. You may believe that any new problem or symptom will be enough to push you over the edge. And fear of falling apart can easily lead to panic: an out-of-control feeling that can actually make this happen.

So get hold of yourself. Pinpoint those particularly difficult things and get help in dealing with them. Don't wait, and don't project a false sense of bravado. If you feel yourself nearing the edge, get someone to help you steady yourself. Discuss your fears. Once you have shared them, you may see things a little more clearly. You may be able to cope with greater strength, knowing that you're not alone. And once you're back in control, your fear will disappear.

What Professional Treatments Are Available?

In some cases, using the techniques we've discussed will bring a sufficient degree of control. However, there may be times when you need additional help. Let's look at the types of treatments that are available.

MEDICATION

Medication is one means of treating intense fears or panic. The medications are designed to block whatever is biochemically contributing to the onset or exacerbation of panic. However, keep in mind that although certain drugs may be beneficial in dealing with panic attacks, they may be inappropriate for some of the lesser fears associated with endometriosis. If you feel that medication may be the answer for you, be sure to speak to your doctor. You'll also want to make sure that any medications prescribed for anxiety or panic are compatible with your endometriosis treatment. (For more information on medications, see chapter 13.)

BEHAVIOR THERAPY

Because fear or panic may lead to additional anxieties and phobias, psychological techniques involving behavior therapy may be quite helpful. For example, techniques such as systematic desensitization, discussed earlier in this chapter, can be very effective in reducing phobias. A qualified therapist should be able to help you better cope with your fears using this technique.

PSYCHOTHERAPY

Because intense fear or panic may throw you out of control, you may require professional intervention—especially if these attacks have been occurring often. Don't feel that you are weak if you decide to consult a professional. After all, your goal is to feel better, right? So if you're having difficulty resolving some of these problems yourself, isn't it good to know that there are experts who can help you regain control?

A Fearless Summary

Although many different fears have been discussed in this chapter, we probably haven't covered all of the ones you could possibly experience. In addition, the coping suggestions offered certainly don't include all possible ways of dealing with fear.

Anticipate that you will fear certain things from time to time. Not only is it okay to be scared, it's normal. Some fears will return. Also remember that the most important thing is to overcome these fears so that they don't overwhelm you.

You're working on recognizing your fears, right? For some of them, you're modifying your behavior. For others, you're modifying your thinking. Soon you will feel more in control. As this happens, you'll notice your fears begin to diminish. That doesn't mean that they'll all go away. But as you work on them, they'll at least lessen in intensity, and you'll feel better knowing that you can handle whatever comes along.

CHAPTER SEVEN

Anger

Gina, age 42, was furious. She was tired of the pain and the medical visits. She was sick of hearing that there was nothing her doctor could do to cure endometriosis. From her doctor to her husband, practically everyone who went near her received an earful! Was Gina angry? You bet your eardrums she was!

In general, people with any chronic medical problem may be angry. It is certainly very common to feel intense anger when you have endometriosis. But because anger results in the buildup of physical energy that needs to be released—in other words, stress—it's important to learn how to cope with this emotion.

Just what is anger? When you have a desire or goal in mind and something interferes with efforts to reach it, this can be very frustrating. A feeling of tension and hostility may result, which is anger.

You may feel anger toward the endometriosis itself, toward your own body, or toward religious beliefs, family, friends, or the medical profession. Virtually anybody may be a target of your anger during your experience with endometriosis. Sometimes it is even an outward manifestation of deeper emotional feelings that are more difficult to express, such as helplessness and frustration.

Are There Different Types of Anger?

To better deal with anger, it helps to know that there are three different ways it can be experienced.

The first type of anger is rage—the expression of violent, uncontrolled anger. If Gina was feeling upset about her endometriosis and a friend told her that she shouldn't get so "worked up" all the time, you can imagine how angry Gina might become. Gina's anger might even lead her to say or do things that would possibly affect her friendship. This is probably the most intense anger you can experience.

The second type of anger is resentment. This feeling is usually kept inside. What if Gina listened to her friend's well-meaning comments, smiled, and said nothing, but was seething inside? This is resentment—a growing, smoldering feeling of anger, directed toward a person or object but often internalized. Resentment tends to sit uncomfortably within you and can do even more physiological and psychological damage than rage.

The third type of anger is indignation, a more appropriate, positive type of anger. Unlike rage, it is released in a controlled, assertive way. If Gina had responded to her friend's comments by stating that she appreciated the concern but would prefer no advice at this point, this would have been an expression of indignation.

Obviously, these three types of anger can occur in combination and in many different ways. Understanding this can help you identify and cope with this powerful emotion when it does occur.

What Causes Anger?

There are, of course, lots of things that can make you angry. You may get angry if you feel that the prescribed treatment isn't helping your endometriosis. You may get angry if you have to wait to see your doctor. Or you may become angry if you feel that your family is not sympathetic to your condition.

Thoughtless comments from others can cause anger, as well. If you sense that someone is taking advantage of you, forcing you to do something against your will, anger may result. If you do not have the ability or confidence to say "no" when friends ask for a favor, this, too, can create feelings of anger—especially if you are too fatigued to complete even your own tasks!

In addition to these causes, there is one more. How about endometriosis—the disease you have? Aren't you angry about this? Knowing your feelings is important, because you must become aware of anger before you can deal with it. Unfortunately, resolving your anger won't make your endometriosis go away. Nor should you think that you would stop being angry if your endometriosis were cured. Neither attitude will help.

In their anger over having endometriosis, one of the most common questions women ask is, "Why me?" This question suggests that having this disease is unfair, or that someone or something is somehow to blame. Again, it's important to realize that in this case, anger is not helpful—that asking "Why me?" will not benefit you in any way. It's far better to ask yourself what you can do about it now.

It is important to realize that anger exists uniquely in the mind of each angry individual. It is a direct result of your thoughts, not of events. An event in and of itself does not make you angry. Rather, your anger is caused by your interpretation of the event—the way you think or feel about it. This is a very important point, one we discuss in much more detail a little bit later, in the section "How Can You Cope with Anger?"

How Does Anger Affect Your Body?

When you are angry, a number of physiological responses occur. Your breathing becomes more rapid, your blood pressure increases (you may feel as if your blood is "boiling"), and your heart begins to pound. Your face may get "hot," and your muscles become tense. You may also feel stronger when angry. The more intense the anger, the greater this feeling of power. In fact, you may be able to remember a time when you were so angry that you almost felt you had superhuman strength.

Anger is a form of energy. The more physical energy that builds up in the body due to anger, the more essential it is to release it. This energy cannot be destroyed. So if it is not released in some constructive manner, it will eventually come out in another, less desirable way.

Imagine the energy from anger as a stick of dynamite about to explode. If you diffuse it, some damage may occur when it explodes, but it won't hurt you as much as it would if you swallowed it to keep others from getting hurt. Obviously, the ideal solution is to neither throw nor swallow the dynamite but to defuse it.

Extreme anger usually passes quickly. If, however, the anger lasts for a long period of time, it can have physically damaging effects on the body. You've probably heard about some of the physical problems that can result from not releasing anger, such as hypertension, diarrhea, and headaches. Well, anger can also exacerbate existing medical problems and make the symptoms of endometriosis more severe. It's just not good for your body.

How Does Anger Affect Your Mind?

Anger is usually experienced as a very unpleasant feeling. However, there may be times that it almost feels good to be angry, probably because of the sense of power or strength you may experience. Sometimes anger may become so extreme that you want to explode. You may feel that if you can't punch, kick, or hit something—to get rid of the anger in some way—you will lose control. Hopefully this angry energy can be released without causing damage to another person, property, or yourself. If, when you finally calm down, you find that you have done something destructive, you may become angry all over again. Or you may experience another negative emotion, such as guilt.

Is Anger Good or Bad?

Is anger ever good or constructive? "Avoid anger at all costs," many say, "because nothing good can come of it." But this is true only if you don't deal with anger properly. Anger can, indeed, be dangerous if it's kept inside or released in inappropriate ways.

Remember that stick of dynamite? What an explosive example! If anger is released in destructive ways, it can cause problems in relationships—to say the least! It can also aggravate your endometriosis. Does this mean that anger can make your condition worse? Well, what if you're so angry at somebody—perhaps your doctor or an overprotective friend—that you don't follow your treatment program, or you do more than you should? "I'll show them," you say.

And then you go on to exhaust yourself. In this case, anger is obviously harmful, but only because you've turned it against yourself.

How can anger be constructive? First, it can be an indication that something is wrong—something that needs attention. Second, it can motivate you to deal more actively with life's problems. Anger can give you a feeling of power or strength, of confidence or assertiveness. We're not saying that you should break dishes or have someone slap you in order to make you angry enough to solve your problems! What we *are* saying is that anger can be positive and, if used correctly, can help you find solutions to real problems.

Some Different Reactions to Anger

Marlene, a 38-year-old teacher, was having a hard time with her husband. He was trying to show his concern by relieving her of some responsibilities around the house. But most days she felt well enough to continue doing her household chores, and she wanted to be treated as normally as possible. She wanted to be the one to determine what she could and could not do. But Marlene's husband didn't see this, and Marlene was running out of patience. Let's look at three ways in which this situation might be handled.

THE "JUST IGNORE IT" APPROACH

If you feel overwhelmed by the intensity of your anger and fear that you could completely lose control, you may do whatever you can to avoid the experience. This might include pushing any angry thoughts out of your mind, no matter how important the issue.

So rather than just focusing on household responsibilities, Marlene could think about other activities and try not to show her resentment. Or she could try to appease her husband and agree with everything he said. This would at least be temporarily effective in helping Marlene to cope. In the long run, however, you can see that this would not be the best way for her to deal with anger—by bottling it up.

THE "TAKE POWER" APPROACH

Maybe you enjoy the flow of energy and strength that comes from being angry. You may find that when you're angry, you are best able to assert yourself and get things done.

Marlene might know that if smothered once too often, she would explode. If she likes the feeling of power she gets from anger, perhaps she wants the chance to say, "Honey, if you treat me that way once more, I'll take these books and . . . !" If you enjoy this feeling, it's possible that you may even provoke situations to make yourself angry. Perhaps you've heard of professional basketball or tennis players who psyche themselves up before a confrontation with an opponent. For them, getting angry is the best preparation for a successful performance!

THE "TAKE ACTION" APPROACH

It's possible to see anger as a necessary, though unpleasant, part of life. You know that there will be times when you'll be angry, whether you like it or not. But you can choose to deal with both your anger and the situation that's causing it as effectively as possible.

For example, Marlene knows that she's not happy being angry, and she might decide to speak to her husband and help him understand her emotional needs. In this case, even if Marlene failed to persuade her husband to understand her need to assume most of her normal household responsibilities, she would at least have the satisfaction of knowing that she did something about her feelings.

Your own reaction to anger is unique. It may also change from time to time. For instance, sometimes you may accept anger and almost value it as a motivator. At other times you may attempt to push it away. Marlene might enjoy expressing her anger. But if she didn't want to hurt her husband or upset the rest of the family, she might choose to have a calm discussion rather than shattering everyone's eardrums with an explosive confrontation.

Of course, how you react to your emotions now is probably similar to the way you reacted in the past. If you have always dealt with problems in a generally positive, constructive manner, you will probably deal with new problems in the same way. On the other hand, if you have had difficulty handling stress in the past, you may also have problems now. But remember that you can learn how to effectively cope with anger, just as Marlene did.

How Can You Cope with Anger?

You've now begun to realize that anger can be constructive. Hopefully, the information you've read so far has been encouraging. But what, specifically, can you do to cope with your own anger?

Because anger is such a complex emotion, and because there are so many things that cause it, there are no simple answers. (Sorry about that!) Does this mean that there is nothing anybody can do about anger? No. You can do a lot to reduce your feelings of anger and to handle them more efficiently, comfortably, and safely.

First, of course, you must be able to admit that you're angry (i.e., recognize it), and figure out *why*. Once you've pinpointed the source of your anger, you may be able to defuse it or, if that's not possible, to find an acceptable outlet. Let's take a look at each of these strategies.

There are two steps involved in recognizing anger: admitting it exists and identifying the source.

STEP ONE: ADMIT THAT YOU'RE ANGRY

The first step in dealing with anger is to recognize that you're angry in the first place. As simple as this may sound, many people cannot take this first step. They may deny it, or they may rationalize their feelings or behavior using other explanations.

Do you feel that being angry is a sign of weakness? If so, you may not admit that you're angry—perhaps not even to yourself. You may feel that there is no appropriate reason to be angry and that it is a childish reaction. But, as with anything else, in order to change something, you have to first recognize that it exists.

How can you tell if you're angry? If you feel very tense (jumping at the sound of the telephone) or find yourself reacting with impulsiveness (slamming down the phone when you get a wrong number and storming out of the house) or become hostile (cursing at your neighbor for leaving a speck of garbage on your lawn), chances are that you're angry. Don't be afraid to recognize it—now you know that this is the first step in dealing with it.

STEP TWO: IDENTIFY THE SOURCE OF YOUR ANGER

The second step in dealing with anger is trying to identify its source. Where did the anger originate? What is contributing to it? What events have led to these feelings of anger?

For one thing, as we mentioned earlier in the chapter, you could certainly be angry because you have endometriosis. At times, you might be angry at your physician, whether it's justified or not. You may be angry because you feel so out of control. In some cases, the events leading to an angry reaction may be quite obvious; in other cases, it may be hard to pinpoint the cause. Keep probing—you will eventually find the source of the problem.

Take the case of Lisa, a 27-year-old attorney. Lisa awakened one bright, cheerful morning to the singing of birds outside her bedroom. Instead of feeling happy and carefree, however, she felt angry. At first, she couldn't figure out why she felt this way on such a beautiful day. Finally, after giving the matter some more thought, she remembered that she was trying a case in front of a hostile judge—something she dreaded. She wished her mood matched the weather a little bit better!

So it's necessary to explain to yourself *why* you're angry. Why is this step important? Because you need to decide whether or not the anger you're feeling is realistic. If necessary, write down what you think is making you feel this way. Be honest when recording your thoughts, regardless of how violent or profane they may be! Rich, colorful language can be helpful in releasing your feelings and will ultimately allow you to control your anger. Try to examine your thoughts objectively, the way someone else might look at them. If, like Lisa, you recognize that your reasons are understandable, this alone may help you deal with your feelings. Your next step will be to decide how you can best handle them.

Now, depending on the situation, you can either defuse your anger or find an appropriate outlet for it. Read on to see how each of these techniques can work for you!

DEFUSE YOUR ANGER

In the past, many believed—incorrectly—that there were only two possible ways to deal with anger: to keep it inside or let it out. But what about a third possibility? Remember when we talked about defusing that stick of dynamite? Your anger is a result of the way you think! In your mind, you're interpreting events in a way that makes you angry. So if you can change the way you interpret things and reorganize your thinking patterns, you can actually stop creating the anger that you feel. Is this really possible? Well, if something happened that made you angry, would everybody in the world be angry because of it? No. Only you would feel this way. Others might not be angry because their interpretation of the event would be different. Let's look at some of the ways that you can defuse your anger *before* it becomes a problem.

Watch Mental Movies

When you become angry, you frequently have all kinds of pictures in your head—images of what's making you angry and of how you'd like to deal with your feelings. These "mental movies" can help you defuse your anger.

For example, imagine that you're in tremendous pain, and very tired. Your friend calls to tell you that her car has broken down. Could you please pick her up? When you tell her that you are really too uncomfortable to go out, she says something about how she can never depend on you for anything. This is a friend? You become irate. At that moment, ask your friend to hold on, close your eyes, and imagine all the abusive things you'd like to say to her. Then imagine the shocked expression on her face. By using this mental imagery, you'll probably be able to complete the phone call without destroying a friendship. You may even smile or laugh as you think about the scenes playing through your mind.

Nan was quite annoyed with her son, Pete. Whenever she asked for his help around the house, he was grouchy and uncooperative. Just before Nan was about to explode, she remembered the mental movie technique and imagined herself clobbering Pete every time he talked back to her. This helped to rid Nan of the intense, angry feelings that were making her crazy, and allowed her to deal with Pete more constructively. Nan was lucky in that she was eventually able to enlist her son's help. She even made a deal with him—she would let him watch football games without interfering as long as he agreed to help her. But even if Nan realized that she would not be able to change her son's behavior, that very realization would have been constructive. How? It would have allowed Nan to move on and seek solutions that didn't require Pete's help. (For more information on dealing with others, see chapter 19.)

Picture a Big Red Stop Sign

Another technique that can help you to control your anger is "thought stopping." Remember: It is the thoughts in your mind that are making you angry—the thoughts you have when you interpret an event. So when you find that angry thoughts have come into your head, picture a big red stop sign. Seeing that picture in your mind will serve as a momentary distraction. Then concentrate on something you enjoy. This can be a peaceful, relaxing scene; a type of food you like; or a favorite movie or television program. Whatever you choose, you will divert your thinking and give your anger a chance to dissipate. You could also participate in a pleasant activity—reading a book, taking a walk, or taking a relaxing bath, for instance. Any of these activities should help defuse your anger.

Change Your Requirements

At times, you may have specific requirements—particular ways that you want certain things to occur. When these needs are not met, you may feel angry. Modifying your demands can help you cope with your anger.

Let's say that you're not feeling well and decide to call your doctor. The answering service tells you that she is not in the office and that you should get a return call within half an hour. After forty-five minutes, the doctor has not yet returned your call, and you are fuming. Why? Because your requirement of having your call returned within thirty minutes was not met.

What can you do? Revise your expectations. Tell yourself that you would have liked a call within thirty minutes, but that your doctor may be in surgery, with another patient, in transit, or simply unable to get to a phone. You'll be satisfied if you get a call at her earliest convenience. By modifying your requirement, you'll feel less angry.

Another way to benefit from this technique is to write down your expectations. Then try to revise them with new, more flexible ones. This may help you see your requirements in a more objective light.

Put Yourself in the Other Person's Shoes

One of the best ways of dealing with anger toward another person is to try and understand exactly what he or she is feeling, wants, or is saying. This will help you accept the behavior and deal with it more constructively. Perhaps just as important, this technique can help you understand how that other person will feel if he or she is the target of an abusive release of anger.

Judy always got angry when her boyfriend insisted that they go out for dinner when he got home from work, especially if she was in pain and the last thing on her mind was food. Judy knew that she had to find a better way to handle her anger. So rather than exploding, she imagined how disappointed he was because, after all, he loved trying new restaurants and going out with her. Judy's new understanding let her defuse her anger and explain why she couldn't always accompany him, even though she wished she felt like going.

LET YOUR ANGER OUT

We have now discussed a number of ways to control your thinking and improve your ability to interpret events to keep your anger from growing. But these techniques might not always be successful. What if there are times when you remain angry? How can you deal with anger in a constructive way when you just can't defuse it? Fortunately, there are two possibilities. Let's see what these are.

Talk, Don't Bite

Obviously, it is much more desirable to discuss an issue constructively than to have an angry exchange of heated words, accomplishing nothing. In most cases, anger arises when you have a conflict or problem with another person. For this reason, it can be very helpful to learn ways to negotiate a solution. Remember that a heated argument—fighting fire with fire—is not the answer. Instead, you want to put out the fire—by reducing the heatedness of the argument.

How can you do this? Try complimenting the person, or looking for positive things that person is saying. Yes, you can do this even though you're angry. This will work in two ways. First, it will probably surprise the person. How will this help? Well, part of what fuels the fire of anger is your anticipation of the other person's anger. So by catching that person off guard, and thereby preventing an angry reaction, you will reduce this fuel. Second, by focusing on words or thoughts that are more constructive, you will calm yourself rather than letting your anger grow. And once you're calm, you'll be able to quietly state your feelings.

Let's take our earlier example in which you became upset by your friend's demands to provide her with a ride. Instead of blowing up and telling her how inconsiderate she is, say that she was right to call you—that you're glad she thought of you. But then tell her that, as much as you would like to do this favor for her, you are not physically able to do it. Regardless of what she says, keep looking for a positive way to respond, and continue to calmly indicate that you don't feel well. Eventually, you'll get your point across. Although she may not be too happy about it—she may even become angry—you will have resolved a problem constructively.

Write Out Your Anger

There are times when something or someone makes you so angry that you feel as if you're going to explode. You recognize the need to release these feelings because they're damaging to you, but you don't have the confidence to speak up. This would be a great time to write an angry letter. Writing can be a constructive way of diffusing this intense anger, without damaging any relationships in the process. For example, you could write to your doctor, your partner, your neighbor, the medical profession, the "powers above," even your endometriosis—virtually anyone, real or not, with whom you feel angry. But remember that for this technique to work best, *don't* let anyone see your letter! After you finish pouring your venom onto paper, destroy it. You'll be destroying some of your anger at the same time!

Find a Physical Release for Your Anger

In general, one of the best outlets for releasing angry energy is physical activity. But what if this is not an option, because of endometriosis, your age, or any other reason? Fortunately, there are solutions.

Some people find that they can release the physical energy from anger by *watching* things! For example, watching a game show may help you to release anger by "getting into" the activities you're viewing. Or you might try watching an emotionally draining movie. You may become so totally absorbed that your built-up energy is released through worry, fear, or excitement. A book that allows you to identify with the characters can be beneficial as well—especially if the characters themselves release anger.

Believe it or not, another common and very effective outlet for anger is crying. We're sure you've heard about the therapeutic effects of a good cry. Although this technique is not for everyone, if your anger has built up to the point of uncontrollable crying, this can be a great way to let it out. (Of course, you may scare the daylights out of your family. But just tell them you read about it here!)

Some people like to count to 10 when angry. This may distract you from what is causing you to feel this way and give you a chance to calm down and think about it more constructively. Try counting out loud and expressing your feelings through facial expressions and tone of voice. Count to a thousand, if necessary!

An Anger-Free Summary

It is important to remember that events alone do not make you angry; what does is how you think and interpret these events. And since it is your thinking that makes you angry, you are responsible for feeling this way. So you must be responsible and help yourself cope with anger—or, at least, reduce it to a more manageable level.

The best way to handle anger is to remain in control, so that it doesn't build up—to restructure your thinking so that your emotions don't get out of hand. But if anger does build, remember that when channeled and used constructively, it can be beneficial. And when this isn't possible, you can defuse or release your anger in a harmless way.

CHAPTER EIGHT

Guilt

Have you ever felt guilty? Many women who have endometriosis say that they have. In fact, family members may feel guilt, as well.

Certainly, it is a very unpleasant feeling. Take the case of Arlene, a 29-year-old mother of two. Before her pain was so severe, one of Arlene's favorite activities was cross-country skiing with her children. Then her doctor suggested she try less strenuous activities when she was having pain. Arlene felt guilty because she stopped participating in an activity that she knew her children enjoyed. In fact, she felt she was being a bad mother. Was it hard for her to cope with this guilt? You bet! But Arlene didn't have to be a victim of this emotion. Let's first take a look at what leads to guilty feelings, and then we'll explore some techniques you can use to help overcome them. After all, you want to do everything possible to make yourself feel better, and it's hard to feel good when you're feeling guilty!

What Are the Two
Components of Guilt?

Feelings of guilt usually have two components. The first is the sense of *wrong-doing*—the notion that you have either done something wrong or have neglected to do something. The second component is the feeling of *badness* that results from this self-blame. It's this factor that's the true culprit! When you feel bad about doing something wrong, this is normal and understandable. But when you start telling yourself that you are a bad person, guilt follows.

What Causes Guilt?

There are a lot of things related to your endometriosis that might make you feel guilty, even though there's probably no validity to any of them. For example, maybe you're concerned that something you did actually caused your endometriosis. Perhaps you feel guilty because you didn't take care of yourself properly, perhaps waiting too long before going to the gynecologist. You could feel that if it weren't for certain actions—or lack of actions—on your part, you would not be in this situation. Or you may feel guilty simply because you are not able to find any rational reason for the disease. Therefore, you blame yourself.

You may also feel guilty if you think that you're complicating matters for your family as a result of your endometriosis. You may worry that you won't be capable of doing what is expected of you. You may feel guilty about letting yourself down or about disappointing others, whether family, friends, or colleagues. Guilt may also result because you are jealous of others who do not have endometriosis.

Perhaps others have told you that your feelings have no rational basis, that you're not at fault. Unfortunately, this may not eliminate guilt. Why? Because your feelings may have nothing to do with what others say or think. Remember: your guilt comes from your own beliefs that you are a bad person.

Obviously, guilt can be a destructive emotion. It can drain you physically and emotionally and can undermine your efforts to cope successfully with endometriosis. Fortunately, there's plenty you can do to improve your outlook.

How Can You Cope with Guilt?

Regardless of the cause of your guilt, and whether or not it is a new or long-standing problem for you, there are a number of strategies that can help you reduce or eliminate this unpleasant and harmful emotion. Let's take a look at some of the best ways.

FIND THE SOURCE OF YOUR GUILT

In order to successfully cope with guilt, you must first focus on what led to the guilty feelings in the first place. Sometimes just by pinpointing the source of this emotion, you can greatly reduce or even eliminate it.

First, ask yourself if you have actually done something wrong. If you really believe that this is true, then ask yourself if your behavior was really so terrible. In Arlene's case, she felt guilty because her endometriosis restricted her activities. Does that make sense? Did she make it happen? Of course not. So identify the cause of your guilt and examine the wrongdoing you think you committed. You will probably find either that you are not responsible for the wrong action, or that it was really not terrible enough to justify feeling so guilty!

Sometimes people feel guilty about thoughts or desires rather than specific actions or behaviors. Recognize the difference between feeling guilty over a thought and feeling guilty over an action. Then, once you've identified the thought that's making you feel like a bad person, change it. Learn to talk to yourself in a positive way. Look at thoughts objectively and constructively.

Monica, a 39-year-old receptionist, felt angry about her endometriosis. She was also extremely lonely because, to her, no one seemed to understand what she was experiencing. It occurred to Monica that she would feel less isolated if her roommate and best friend, Jane, also had endometriosis. This thought, of course, caused Monica feelings of great guilt. How could she possibly wish endometriosis on her best friend? Gradually, though, Monica came to realize that she did not really want her friend to have endometriosis; she was simply trying to deal with her own loneliness and anger. By understanding this, and by using strategies to better handle her emotions, Monica not only eliminated her guilt but also improved her whole outlook.

But what if you feel guilty and simply can't remember what you were thinking or doing that made you feel this way? How can you use all the great thought-changing ideas we're going to talk about if you can't identify the ones you want to change? Good question! In order to pinpoint these "target" thoughts or behaviors, you might want to keep a brief written log of feelings or activities that may be causing your guilt. Once you have recorded them, you can begin to determine the root of the problem and then think about what changes might improve the situation.

Betty, age 44, had been feeling increasingly guilty but didn't really know why. By keeping a log she noticed that, besides complaining of pain all the time, she had been arriving late to work on a regular basis. She wasn't aware of how frequently she had been late—and she had always been so proud of her punctuality! The log helped her see that she needed to change her morning routine in order to be more punctual. As she worked on this problem, her guilt lessened.

TALK IT OVER

It's very important to discuss your feelings about having endometriosis with others who may be affected by it. Share your concerns, and try to figure out solutions to any problems that exist.

Joann, a single woman of 33, had enjoyed a very active social life before her endometriosis pain became so intense. In addition to going out on weekends, she and her best friend, Eleanor, would play doubles in a tennis league at least two or three times a week. Now, because of the pain of endometriosis, all too often Joann had to cancel her activities. She just couldn't do as much as she used to. Naturally, Joann wasn't happy about her new limitations. In addition, she felt extremely guilty about holding her friend back.

Fortunately, Joann had the good sense to sit down with Eleanor and discuss the situation. Together they decided that until Joann regained some of her strength, she would rest at home while Eleanor continued to play tennis with other partners. To end their discussion on a positive note, together they decided that when she felt better they would take a vacation. Joann felt better knowing that her limitations would not prevent her friend from enjoying her favorite activities. Joann also had something to look forward to—a fun trip.

TURN YOUR THOUGHTS AROUND

Is there anything you can do about the negative thoughts that lead to guilt— those thoughts that make you feel that you're a bad person? One helpful thing to do is try to restructure your thinking to make it more positive and guilt-free.

For example, let's say that you feel guilty because you believe that you're not being a good mother. Ask yourself if you've ever done anything that a good mother might do. Just about every mom can name many things! This type of thinking will begin to eliminate your "bad mother blues." The idea is to turn your mind's negative thoughts into reasonable, positive ones. This way, the feeling of guilt will not become a stranglehold!

REEVALUATE YOUR GOALS

Because of the pain and fatigue she suffered as a result of her endometriosis, Carla, a 40-year-old mother of three, had to stay home frequently from her job. As a result, she earned less money and couldn't provide all of the luxuries that she and her family had previously enjoyed. Feeling guilty, Carla tried to push herself harder to increase her earnings, which in turn made her feel worse physically. Obviously, Carla was not coping well with her guilt. Instead, she was allowing it to affect her health.

Do you, like Carla, see a difference between the way you are doing something and the way you think you *should* be doing it? If so, you are probably feeling guilty! How can you work this out? Can you work harder or do more? If you can, and it's appropriate for you to do so, then you've solved your problem. If not, try examining your day-to-day goals for working and living. Ask yourself if these goals are practical, considering what you can and cannot do because of your endometriosis.

When evaluating your goals, you may find that among the most common causes of guilt are thoughts containing the word "should." "Should" is a dirty word! Carla thought that she "should" have been able to work harder and earn more money. Other "should" thoughts might include: "I should have been able to finish cleaning that room today" or "I really should be taking my kids to the park today." These "should" thoughts imply that you must be just about perfect and right on top of everything. Naturally, you will become upset whenever you fall short of your "should." But are you to blame when "should" thoughts establish goals that are unrealistic—goals you may not be able to fulfill? Obviously, the answer is no!

In order to feel better and reduce guilt, reword your thoughts to eliminate the word "should." Use less demanding ones. Say, "It would be nice if I could finish that task today, but I can't," rather than "I should finish that task today." If you have trouble changing the wording of your "should" thoughts, try asking yourself, "Why should I . . . ?" or "Who says I should . . . ?" or "Where is it written that I should . . . ?" This may help you decide whether you are setting up impossible requirements for yourself and help you reduce your guilt.

Let's say, for example, that you are thinking of having a party because all of your friends have invited you to get-togethers. Ask yourself why you should feel obligated to reciprocate. Is it because the "Party Rulebook" tells you that if you don't have a party, your friendship license will be revoked? Is it because if you don't have a party, your friends—some friends!—won't invite you to their homes anymore? As you think of some realistic answers to these questions, it will be easier to realize that you don't have to entertain. Although it would be nice, it would be more sensible to wait until you're feeling better.

Another way to eliminate guilt feelings over "should" thoughts is to take more pride in what you *can* do rather than focusing on things you feel you should do but can't. Although most people hate hearing "Things could be worse," in the case of endometriosis this may be quite true. If you concentrate on what you are able to do rather than the negative, your feelings of guilt will diminish and you'll feel a lot better. Changing your thinking will also help you reduce the perceived gap between what is real and what you feel "should" be—which is what led to your guilty feelings in the first place.

ESCAPE FROM ESCAPE BEHAVIOR

Sometimes people who fail to cope with their guilt act in negative ways to hide from their feelings. They may also indulge in "escape" behaviors, such as drinking or excessive sleeping. This behavior does not confront problems head-on but instead attempts to push them away.

As you may have already guessed, the first step toward improvement is to look past the escape behavior and identify what is causing the guilt. Then consider what can be done to rectify the problem. At the same time, try to eliminate the escape behavior, recognizing that this activity is not improving your situation in any way. If you have difficulty doing this by yourself—or, for that matter, in identifying the root of the problem—by all means consider working with a supportive professional. You're worth it!

It is possible, of course, that there is no clear-cut way to eliminate the situation or feelings that have led to your guilt. But don't give up. Instead, look for partial answers. This may not be as desirable as finding complete solutions, but it can still help reduce your guilt and make you feel better about yourself.

A Final Guiltless Thought

Guilt is a very destructive emotion—one that can interfere with your success in coping with endometriosis by lowering your self-image and exhausting your emotional resources. Becoming aware of how guilt develops, pinpointing the source of your guilt, and changing your thinking to be more positive and realistic, can help decrease or eliminate this feeling. This should leave you with more energy to successfully cope with your endometriosis.

CHAPTER NINE

Stress

Stress! Every time you turn around, you either read or hear about stress. What exactly is it? Stress is a response that occurs in your body. It is a form of energy—a normal reaction to the demands of everyday life. It helps you mobilize your strength to deal with different events and circumstances.

Many things occur each day that require you to adapt; these are known as *stressors*. The change that takes place in your body when a stressor provokes you is known as the *stress response*.

Stress can play a role in exacerbating virtually any medical problem, and endometriosis is no exception. On the other hand, some women with endometriosis worry that maybe not managing their stress appropriately caused their disease. This simply is not true.

Chances are you've been feeling a lot of pressure lately and would be a lot happier if you could lower your stress level. So let's learn more about stress—what causes it, how it can affect you, and, most important, how you can learn to cope with it.

What Are the Symptoms of Stress?

Your body will tell you when the stress you're experiencing is excessive. What might you feel? Physical signs include sweaty palms, heart palpitations, tightness of the throat, fatigue, nausea, diarrhea, or headaches—among other things. Depression, anxiety, anger, frustration, or simply a vague uneasiness are just a few possible emotional reactions. Of course, endometriosis causes many of the same symptoms, so it might be hard to separate the two. So what is most important is to tune into both your body and your mind, and then you'll know when you can benefit from stress-reduction techniques.

How Does Stress Affect You?

The effects of stress—much like the effects of depression, discussed in chapter 5—are not isolated problems. Instead, they are part of a complex response that can involve both your body and your emotions.

HOW STRESS AFFECTS YOUR BODY

Stress is a natural survival response. It occurs within the body whenever you feel threatened by thoughts or external pressures.

Stress can manifest itself in many ways. When you are in a stressful situation, your circulatory system works faster and blood is pushed rapidly toward different parts of the body—particularly to the protective organs and systems raising your blood pressure. Because the blood supply has been diverted to other organs, digestion is usually slowed. Stress also constricts the blood vessels, increases heart rate, and produces other physiological manifestations— all instantaneously!

What else can occur? Trembling and perspiring are very common reactions. Your face may flush. Then you feel a surge of adrenaline flowing through your body. Your mouth may become dry, or you may feel nauseated. Your breathing may become more rapid and shallow, or your heart may begin to pound. Your muscles may become tight, leading to headaches or cramps. Sounds wonderful, doesn't it?

So when you experience stress, your body prepares itself physiologically to counter any threat to its survival. Why? Well, perhaps you've heard of the *fight-or-flight syndrome.* When an animal feels threatened, it prepares to either fight or run away. You will never see an animal standing there, scratching its head, and thinking about how to best handle the situation! Even though we have the ability to think and reason, we also experience the fight-or-flight syndrome, which causes the secretion of many different hormones and tenses the muscles in preparation for battle. If the response does involve physical action—fight or flight—the hormones are utilized as they should be and the muscles exercised, with energy being appropriately released. However, if there is no physical exertion—if you *think* instead of taking action—the energy that was mobilized may not be released in the most appropriate way. This may explain why, after a period of stress when no action was taken, you feel exhausted just the same.

When does stress lead to physical problems? When you can't respond in a way that eliminates it, the stress continues unabated—and so do its symptoms. If you are not able to relieve the stress, you end up causing even more stress, creating a vicious cycle. And this can take its toll on your body. If stress is not controlled, it can make your endometriosis worse.

HOW STRESS AFFECTS YOUR MIND

Your emotional response to stress may not be as obvious as your physical response. You may start worrying and fear the next "event." Your attention span is then reduced, and you are less able to concentrate on the task at hand. You may have trouble learning something new and even be afraid to do things. You may withdraw or feel nervous. You may begin to lose confidence in yourself.

As you become nervous and upset, you are likely to notice some unpleasant physical responses you're experiencing, and this may make you feel even more stressed. For example, if you experience shallow, rapid breathing or heart palpitations, your awareness of these reactions may lead to feelings of panic. Most people respond to stress both physically and emotionally, although it is possible to respond in only one way. Don't you have your own "typical" reaction? Maybe you become too jittery and unfocused to concentrate on your job. Perhaps you feel physically ill, with extreme intestinal discomfort, diarrhea, or a throbbing headache. Regardless of what you experience, it's important to learn strategies that will help you cope.

Three Reactions to Stress

We've just discussed how your body and mind respond to stress. But we also want to look at a third type of response—the way you choose to deal with stress.

When a stressful stimulus occurs, you will most likely react in one of three ways. You might not respond at all and either "go with the flow" or become unable to function. You might respond immediately and impulsively without giving thought to whether a better response might be possible. Or you might respond to stressors in a well-planned, organized, and effective manner. If so, you may not even need this chapter! But we recommend that you read on!

Is Stress Good or Bad?

By now, you've probably figured out that stress can be either good or bad. If it gives you extra energy to do the things that you must do to conquer your emotions—then it is good. In fact, a certain amount of stress is normal and necessary. Stress helps you "get your act together" and prepares you to handle your life in the best possible way. But when left unchecked, stress can be highly destructive, draining all of your energy and possibly worsening your endometriosis symptoms or any emotional problems. So while stress can be helpful, this chapter concerns itself with harmful stress—the kind that can hurt you if it goes uncontrolled.

What Causes Stress?

A number of things can act as stressors. Work-related problems, relationship disputes, family deaths, even some positive events—all can cause stress. In this book, we're most concerned with the effects of endometriosis on your life, and this can cause stress in a number of different ways. For example, pain can cause stress. Waiting for test results can cause stress. Concerns about how the endometriosis may affect you can cause stress. Worries about not being able to fulfill family or career responsibilities can cause stress. Wondering if you will ever become pregnant can cause stress. Medication side effects, anticipating surgery, fear of complications, adjustments to dietary changes, and financial and family pressures may also provoke a stress response.

Do events by themselves cause stress? And will the events that cause stress in one person necessarily cause it in another—and to the same degree? As you may have guessed, the answer is no! Why? Because, as we mentioned earlier in the chapter on anger (chapter 7), every person has a unique way of responding. Your reactions depend on a number of things. Your upbringing, your self-esteem, your beliefs about yourself and the world, the way you guide yourself in your thoughts and actions—all of these things help determine your response. How well you feel in control of your life also plays an important role. And your physical and emotional health—as well as your response to others—is also a factor.

To sum up, everyone's method of dealing with stress is unique and individual and depends on a complex combination of thoughts and behaviors. To keep things simple, though, we can view the stress response as dependent on the "chemistry" between two factors. The first factor is the stressor, or the outside pressure. In other words, what is going on around you that is creating a problem? The second factor is your interpretation of the event. The interaction of the stressor and your internal interpretation together determine your response to stress. (Sound familiar? Yes, it's the same "formula" that can be applied to anger, depression, and any other emotion.) The "equation" for the stress response is as follows:

Stressor + Interpretation = Stress Response

This equation has important implications for coping with stress, because it indicates that stress is not solely the result of your environment, endometriosis, or any other factor around you. The way you interpret this stressor is of equal importance. Of course, some stressors would produce a negative response in anybody. What would happen, for example, if somebody pointed a knife at your throat? Calm acceptance or a stress response? Get the point? In many situations, though, you do have the ability to control your reaction.

As you learn to cope with stress, it's important to remember that your mind responds to any threats as though they are real and happening right now. The brain and the nervous system perceive any stressful thoughts or images in your mind as existing in the present, because they do not recognize the difference between past, present, and future. So, you contribute to your body's stress response with your own thoughts and images. This makes it even more important to feed your mind with the best, most beneficial, and most constructive information available.

How Can You Cope with Stress?

Because stress can affect the body and mind in so many ways, learning how to manage it is a very important part of any program for coping with endometriosis. We still don't know the effect that prolonged stress can have on the body's vulnerability to endometriosis. But we do know that it can certainly play a role in exacerbating the unpleasant and often debilitating symptoms. And we also know that endometriosis causes enormous amounts of stress on physical, social, and psychological levels. The good news is that, regardless of how you have handled stress in the past, you can learn effective strategies that will help you effectively deal with it now. These strategies will make you feel more in control, lessening the feelings of panic and increasing your emotional well-being. And because of the mind–body connection, these strategies will also help your body better cope with endometriosis.

Before we look at how you should cope with stress, let's look at what you *shouldn't* do. Smoking, alcohol abuse, the use of inappropriate drugs, and overeating are all common behaviors many individuals use, but they are poor coping strategies. True, these activities will distract you and perhaps delay the effects of the stress, but they can also hurt you and prevent you from coping in a constructive way.

So what should you do? Try to learn new, more appropriate ways of dealing with stress. Relaxation techniques and regular exercise are important components of a stress management program. Thinking more appropriate and positive thoughts is also helpful. But be realistic and remember that while stress can be managed and controlled, it cannot be eliminated. Your focus, then, should be on using some of the following management techniques to help yourself deal better with both its physical and the emotional effects.

USE RELAXATION TECHNIQUES

Because relaxation is incompatible with stress, the best way to start coping is to relax. In fact, relaxation techniques alone may allow you to successfully cope with both the physical and the emotional effects of stress.

Relaxation benefits you in many ways. First, it can give your body a chance to rest and recuperate. And a stronger body can help you deal better with the ravages of stress—and life!—and enable you to derive increased benefits from any other treatments. Relaxation will also help you sleep better and recover from surgery (if you need it) faster. It is pleasurable and will increase your feeling of emotional well-being. And it can give you a powerful sense of reestablishing control over your life despite having a chronic disease.

There are many different types of clinical relaxation techniques, including meditation, autogenics, and deep breathing. You may also want to investigate hypnosis and biofeedback as ways to relax, although they have other uses as well. (See chapter 12 for a full discussion of these and other relaxation techniques.)

One technique that is often successful in combating stress is imagery, a method that can also be used to cope with pain and other problems. Imagery is the process of formulating mental pictures or scenes in order to harness your body's energy and improve your physical or emotional well-being. In this case, of course, you'll want to conjure up images that are relaxing and stress-free.

Denise always became tense in anticipation of her menstrual period, worrying about an increase in pain. She often was so nervous that she found it almost impossible to eat or sleep. Denise was instructed to relax in her favorite chair, dim the lights, and avoid any interruptions. She then imagined herself lying on a blanket at the beach. She felt the warmth of the sun and the caress of a gentle breeze on her legs. She heard the sounds of the waves lapping against the shore, and the familiar call of seagulls. She smelled the salt water and the suntan lotion. Soon, Denise began to relax. She relaxed so well, in fact, that she began to doze.

Of course, you'll want to imagine a scene that is particularly relaxing for you. Denise found the beach especially soothing. You may prefer another image. To make this technique work most effectively, try to make your images multisensory, as Denise did. In other words, imagine not only the sights, but also the smells, the tactile sensations (touch), and the sounds. The more vivid your image, the more helpful it will be. The degree of relaxation you'll experience depends completely on you and how much you practice. You are in control.

PINPOINT THE SOURCE OF YOUR STRESS

Now that you're more relaxed, you're ready to objectively identify your stressors. What, specifically, is causing you to feel stress? Maybe you're having a hard time dealing with the debilitating symptoms of endometriosis. Perhaps you are concerned about the reactions of others. Or you may be at risk of losing your job. Of course, there are many more possibilities.

What if you're unsure what's causing your stress? Try keeping a log. This will allow you to more easily recognize the people, places, and things that have the potential to create stress in your life. If you can't pinpoint which of your many activities are the real culprits, as you keep your log, you might want to use a numerical rating scale, such as the Subjective Units of Disturbance (SUD) Scale. How does it work? Ratings on this scale range from 0 to 100, depending on the amount of stress you're experiencing. Use 100 to represent the most extreme and disturbing stress, and 0 to represent no stress— total and complete relaxation. Then rate your activities, experiences, and thoughts. The ones with the higher SUD numbers are the ones causing you the most tension. (For example, loud music blasting from your neighbor's radio might be rated a whopping 85!)

IDENTIFY YOUR STRESS REACTIONS

Once you have begun identifying your stressors, you'll want to become completely aware of your responses. Are they more physiological or psychological? What parts of your body seem to be the most vulnerable? Does your attention span suffer? Do you get heart palpitations? Do you start losing confidence or feel as if you're "slipping"? As you become more aware of these things, you will develop a complete picture of your own unique stress response. This picture will help you choose the most useful coping strategies for dealing with the events that trigger your stress.

ELIMINATE STRESSORS WHEN POSSIBLE

What's the next step? Once you recognize which stressors are causing the most trouble, try to determine whether or not you can eliminate them. Removing the source of the stress is an obvious and logical way to manage it. For instance, if the task of managing your household expenses is increasing your anxiety, you might have your husband or another family member take over this chore. Obviously, different types of stressors would have to be removed in other ways.

CHANGE YOUR VIEW OF THE STRESSOR

What happens if you can't eliminate the source of your stress? You'll then have to work on your interpretation of the stressors. You might want to use some of the relaxation techniques suggestions discussed in chapter 12 on managing pain. Or you might want to try systematic desensitization, discussed in chapter 6.

Another technique that might help you cope better is *stress inoculation.* How can you be inoculated against stress? Well, you're certainly familiar with the use of inoculations to protect children from such diseases as measles. Exposing a child to the virus or other agent that causes a disorder gradually strengthens the child's immunity to the disorder. Similarly, stress inoculation uses mental rehearsal procedures to help you confront and, gradually, tolerate stressful situations. As we discussed previously, because your mind responds to thoughts and mental images as if they were real and happening right now, thinking about something can be just as stressful as experiencing it. So by learning to cope with a situation in your mind, you can learn to deal with it before it even happens.

Start your stress inoculation process by using whatever relaxation techniques you have found most helpful. Once you have achieved a comfortable level of relaxation, start imagining one of the stressors you've previously identified. As you imagine the stressful scene, recognize any physiological sensations or psychological changes that you may be experiencing.

Jan realized that much of her stress was being caused by the fear that, during an office visit, her doctor would tell her that her endometriosis had worsened. Jan's stress reaction—nausea and a tightening of the throat—would appear whenever she imagined this unpleasant occurrence. So she decided to use stress inoculation to gain control. Repeatedly she imagined herself in the very situation she feared. She visualized the doctor's office. She imagined herself sitting in the chair by the doctor's desk. She actually heard the words she feared. As Jan gradually increased her tolerance of this image, the symptoms of her stress lessened.

Like Jan, whenever you use stress inoculation to visualize and mentally experience a scene, you'll increase your ability to handle that particular stressor and your symptoms will decrease. In other words, your body and mind will be "inoculated," allowing you to tolerate that stressor. One added advantage of using this technique is that you will become more aware of exactly when these tension-producing situations begin to affect you. This will enable you to use your coping strategies sooner, before your body and mind begin suffering from the stress response.

But don't feel that you have to use stress inoculation for every stressor you anticipate experiencing. And don't think you have to deal with every stressor all at once. Work with each scene individually until you feel you've mastered it.

If you have already read the explanation of systematic desensitization found in chapter 6, you may realize that stress inoculation and desensitization are very similar. But there is a difference. In desensitization, the technique of imagining a stressful situation is alternated with the use of relaxation techniques. In stress inoculation, relaxation techniques are employed only at the start of each session. Experimentation will show you which method is best for you.

By the way, you may benefit from a "real-life" stress inoculation simply by listening to the stories of other women with endometriosis. By learning what others have gone through, in support groups, chatrooms, books, or contact networks, you may become desensitized to some of the issues you may face having endometriosis.

USE PHYSICAL STRESS RELIEVERS

Certain physical activities can be a great means of stress control. As long as you are physically able—and enjoy activities—they can be very relaxing. There are a number of activities that you may find help reduce stress and symptoms associated with endometriosis.

Exercise

Exercise is not only a wonderful means of releasing stress but, as you'll learn in chapter 16, can be a very healthy component of any treatment program. Regardless of how endometriosis is affecting you, there is a type of exercise that will help you control your level of stress. Brisk walking, swimming, and dancing, for instance, all allow for the release of tension. Walking your dog every day (or an imaginary one) is fun and good for both of you. If you have any concerns about certain activities, just be sure to get your doctor's approval before beginning.

Keep Busy the Fun Way

Hobbies and other leisure activities are often very effective ways to reduce stress. They can divert your attention from the unpleasant situation and direct it toward something more enjoyable. They may also cause you to feel productive—and a lack of productivity may be one of the stressors giving you problems in the first place! If you don't have a hobby, this is a great time to look into painting, knitting, sculpting—whatever suits your fancy. If you already participate in leisure activities, now you have the perfect reason to indulge yourself whenever you can. Sometimes, just being outside, working in your garden on a beautiful, sunny day, is enough activity to put you in a calm state of mind.

Catch Up on Your Sleep

Another technique for dealing with stress is sleep. Some people have difficulty sleeping when they're experiencing high levels of stress. But when possible, catnaps or even prolonged periods of sleep may help you reduce stress to a more manageable level. After all, you need your rest, anyway! You might want to consider chair pads that provide heat and pulsing massage or that incorporate magnetic technology. These can enhance your sense of well-being, which leads to relaxation and other benefits.

A Stress-Free Summary

What are your goals? Are you trying to gain greater control over your emotions? Do you want to live life more fully? Whatever they are, if stress is keeping you from reaching them, then your stress response is negative. By learning how to control your stress—by eliminating stressors or by modifying your reaction—you'll be far more likely to meet these goals. Just as important, you'll have a head start in coping successfully with endometriosis.

CHAPTER TEN

Other Emotions

The emotions discussed in chapters 5 through 9 are not the only ones you may experience as a result of your endometriosis. What other feelings could concern you? This chapter will discuss four additional emotions that many women with endometriosis have found to be problematic: boredom, envy, loneliness, and grief.

Boredom

Hopefully, by this time, you are not so bored that you have stopped reading! If we've still got your attention, let's talk a little bit about boredom.

What an empty feeling boredom is! It's one of the worst feelings you can possibly experience. It has been said that more problems and tragedies are caused by boredom than by any other single emotion. We bet you never thought of endometriosis as being boring. But it can be, primarily because of the restrictions your condition may impose on you. Many activities that provided enjoyment for you in the past may now be out of reach. You may not even want to bother starting something new, as you may feel that future activities will become too restricted because of your condition.

So what should you do? To begin with, don't let endometriosis cause you to give up on life. Distinguish between what you can do and what you can't. If you do have to curtail some things because of endometriosis, you'll do so. If you have to drop an activity, you'll drop it. But don't eliminate everything that you enjoy doing simply because you feel that you may be unable to finish. How else can you fight the boredom blues? Read on!

TRY NEW ACTIVITIES

If boredom is a problem, you'll certainly want to find ways to add some interest to your life. You may find that the activities you used to enjoy now seem artificial and uninteresting or that you no longer derive any pleasure from them. This sometimes happens as we mature and grow during various stages of life. Don't feel that you must push yourself to enjoy these activities you once enjoyed, as forcing yourself to be amused rarely works. Instead, try to find something new that will make your life more interesting. Remember that preferences change. Be open-minded and try hobbies, sports, travel, or events that never appealed to you before. This time around, they may spark your interest.

LEARN SOMETHING NEW

One of the most effective weapons against boredom is learning. The mind is like a sponge, always thirsty to soak up information and knowledge. Select a potentially interesting topic that you don't know much about. Then go out and learn something about it. You may want to begin by simply going to the library and reading some books on the topic. Or surf the Internet and see what you can find. Perhaps you'd like to enroll in an adult education course. Boredom often disappears once you become involved in something new. As an added benefit, your new pursuit may put you in contact with some interesting new people. And increasing your circle of friends is always a good way to fight boredom.

SET GOALS

Boredom often arises from plodding along with no purpose in life. So one of the best ways to fight it is to always give yourself something to look forward to—a goal. This doesn't mean that you'll never be bored. You may still have to give yourself an occasional kick in the butt to get yourself moving toward those goals. But the promise of some pleasurable activity will make it much easier to keep yourself going.

What kinds of goals might you set? They can be as simple as reading a chapter of a good book, writing a letter, making that phone call you've been thinking about, talking a walk in the park, or meeting somebody special for lunch. Remember that your life is not over! Try to schedule something that will excite you every day. This way, even if part of your day seems boring—because you're involved in household tasks or because you have to rest to build up your strength—you won't give the weeds of boredom a chance to take root!

Envy

You've heard the cliché "The grass is always greener..." If you have endometriosis, you're probably envious of those who don't—of women who feel well and don't experience pain like you do. This is understandable. But envy is still a destructive emotion, because it's a type of self-torture. When you feel envious, you're constantly putting yourself down and comparing your own qualities with the seemingly better qualities of somebody else. You feel inferior. And this can lead to other negative emotions, such as anger or depression.

Envy is often irrational. When you're envious, you want to be like somebody else. You want to have what somebody else has. Does this mean that the other person's life is happier than yours in every way? Stop and think for a moment. I'm sure you can come up with some areas in which your life is better!

What Leads to Envy?

Basically, there are four conditions necessary for envy to occur. First, you must feel deprived in some way. You must feel as if you can't have something that you want or need. We're not talking simply about money, pleasure, or even health! Envy is an intense emotion that involves much more than this. It seems as if your feeling of need lies deep inside.

Second, to experience envy you must feel that another person has something you don't have. Perhaps that person has a bigger house, for instance. Or in the case of a woman who does not have endometriosis, she has "healthy insides"!

Third, you must feel powerless to do anything about this problem. You must think that you are unable to change the circumstances that have made you envious in the first place. This helplessness causes you to become more and more bitter. And this makes you even more envious!

Fourth, there must be a change in the relationship between you and the person you envy. You are no longer simply comparing yourself with that person; you are now fiercely competitive. You may begin to feel that the only reason you don't have what you want is because somebody else has it.

There are two categories of things that may cause you to feel envy. One is tangible—jewelry, cars, homes, and so on. The other type is less tangible—friends, pleasure, or health, for instance. Even though you have endometriosis, you may still have many tangible things such as a car and a nice place to live. You may still have a job. But your medical condition can certainly cause you to feel envious over less tangible things.

MAKE THE BEST OF WHAT YOU HAVE

To rid yourself of this destructive emotion, concentrate on increasing the benefits and pleasures you *can* get out of life. Why worry about comparing yourself with somebody else? How is that going to help you? Sure, you have endometriosis. But that doesn't mean you can't get a lot of enjoyment from life. Set up reasonable goals for yourself, considering what valuable things you *do* have and what you are capable of doing. Remember that you are who you are. Make the best of what your life has to offer.

Loneliness

There is a difference between being alone and being lonely. Being alone simply means that there is no one else with you. This can be either good or bad. But being lonely is always negative. Loneliness is a sad, empty feeling. The result is that you become upset by your awareness of being alone.

WHY ARE YOU LONELY?

Why might you feel lonely? If you can't spend time with your friends like you used to as a result of your pain, you may feel left out. Or you may feel isolated because you think that others don't understand your condition and why you are so frequently in pain. Having endometriosis may also make you feel isolated from other women who are healthy. And you may decide to change some of your relationships just because you're having difficulty dealing with people.

It's hard to be lonely—and not just because it is such an awful feeling. You see, loneliness doesn't just happen; it actually takes effort to make and keep yourself lonely. There are many opportunities to enjoy the company of others. As a result, loneliness usually occurs out of choice rather than by accident. To be really lonely, you must purposely exclude everyone around you from your life. You have to always be on your guard, protecting yourself from the horrible possibility of making new friends!

DO YOU *WANT* TO BE LONELY?

Why would you want to be lonely? There are four possible reasons. First, deep down you may actually enjoy this feeling. In fact, you may enjoy it so much that you refuse to do anything about it. Why? Because you may feel more comfortable alone than in the company of others.

Second, if you're lonely, you may be hard to please. You may feel that you don't want to even bother trying to create new relationships because no one meets all of your requirements.

Third, you may feel that being lonely is unavoidable. You may have resigned yourself to it. In fact, you could be telling yourself right now that this is an unavoidable situation due to your endometriosis!

Fourth, and probably most important, you may be lonely because you're scared. You may be afraid of rejection. You may recall previous relationships that didn't work out the way you wanted and feel that they are simply not worth the hurt and pain or the lengthy explanation that is necessary to educate someone about your disease.

END YOUR LONELY WAYS

Fortunately, whether your loneliness has been plaguing you for some time or is a relatively new problem, there is a light at the end of the tunnel! Recognize what causes your feeling of loneliness. Admit to yourself that you should try to change this destructive emotion. Then do all you can to fight it.

Don't Be a Pusher

The first step in ending loneliness is to stop pushing people away. It's likely that you're giving off unseen vibrations—vibrations telling people that you don't want them around. These vibrations can reduce your number of acquaintances, adding to your feeling of loneliness. This must stop. You have to learn to give off positive vibrations—the type that welcomes others instead of chasing them away. Smile at people. Show interest in what they have to say and let them know that you like being with them.

Make Contact!

Once you start giving off new, more positive vibes, you'll want to make more friends. How can you meet people? One way is by getting involved in an organization. Because you have endometriosis, you may want to contact your local chapter of either the Endometriosis Association or the Endometriosis Research Center. There, you'll meet other women with similar concerns. Besides relieving your loneliness, the members of your group may also share some valuable coping skills. You may even find ways of helping others.

If support groups aren't your cup of tea, try getting involved in a new learning activity or hobby. Take adult education courses, for example. This may help to alleviate loneliness as well as boredom. Invite people to your home. Most important, be receptive to the people you meet. Try to see the good in everyone. Don't reject someone simply because there are a few things about them that you don't like.

If you work at conquering loneliness, you'll feel much better about yourself and your life. This will make living more enjoyable, even with endometriosis. Give yourself and others a chance, and your feelings of loneliness will disappear, regardless of the limitations your condition has placed on you.

Grief

Grief is an unpleasant emotion. And feelings of grief—the mourning over a loss—are common in women with endometriosis, especially at the time of initial diagnosis or after major surgery, such as a hysterectomy. You may also grieve over your inability to have children.

WHY ARE YOU GRIEVING?

People grieve when they're aware that they've lost something of value. Although you may never have consciously thought about how much you valued your insides, you may now. Endometriosis can make you feel that you have changed or that you have lost some physical strength. As a result, you may not like yourself as much and are grieving your damaged self-esteem. If you are used to playing a certain role within your family, and this has been modified because of your endometriosis, you may grieve this loss as well.

Sherry, a 40-year-old account executive, took pride both in the position of responsibility she held in her company and in her income, which helped support her family. Then along came some of the devastating effects of endometriosis. Because Sherry's work was so demanding, with long hours, there was a possibility that she would not be able to continue working in the field she loved so much. Sherry grieved the possible loss of her career.

Grief is not always bad. When this feeling develops, it means that you must work it out before you can adjust to the new situation—in this case, endometriosis.

WORK THROUGH YOUR GRIEF

What can you do about grief? Unfortunately, it cannot be avoided. But by analyzing your grief and working through it, you can get back to the act of living. Sherry had to face the realities of her situation and see how she might take on less demanding work. Only by focusing on the source of her grief and beginning to address these concerns could Sherry begin to feel better.

CRY

How else can you combat grief? Crying can be helpful. This doesn't mean that you should force yourself to sob, but if the tears start welling up, don't stop them. Let your feelings out. Think about what has changed and what will change. Talk it out with the people you trust. Don't avoid the fact that you have endometriosis, as this denial will prevent you from going through the grief process.

Remember that grief is like a deep infection. The only way it can improve is to open it and let what's inside come out, even if it means a good cry. This may be difficult, but eventually the wound will drain and begin to heal. Soon you will exhaust your grief. Then the healing will begin.

Living with endometriosis can involve a number of painful emotions. But it is possible to cope with these emotions—to learn constructive approaches that will eliminate or lessen them and help you live more comfortably and happily. These strategies are just what the doctor—and family and friends—ordered!

PART THREE

Changes in General Lifestyle

CHAPTER ELEVEN

Coping with Lifestyle Changes—an Introduction

Some changes in your lifestyle because of endometriosis are probably inevitable. But remember that throughout life, changes can occur for any number of reasons. If you began a new job, you might have to wake up earlier, commute in a new direction using a different form of transportation, or adjust to a change in salary. And if your new job required you to move, you would have to meet a whole new group of people.

In your case, it's endometriosis that has now changed your life. Although you may think that it will be impossible to ever lead a normal life again, hopefully this isn't true. However, you must make certain changes that will help you lead a comfortable life despite endometriosis. Remember that you want to feel better, enjoy life, and do what you can. These goals are both reasonable and achievable.

To different degrees, endometriosis can affect work, school, family life, sexual activity, social activity, finances, and other aspects of day-to-day living. Be determined to make any necessary changes. But also be aware that you may continually find ways that will improve the way you live. In addition, remember that your lifestyle will, to a large degree, be your own choice. You'll automatically consider many different factors when determining what you want your lifestyle to be.

You may decide to postpone things—to avoid making any changes until you "feel better." But why wait? Why not do what you can right now to improve the quality of your life, even while you're learning to live with endometriosis?

What Changes May Take Place?

Endometriosis can change your lifestyle because of a number of different factors:

- Its effects on your body can cause miscarriages, infertility, limit sexual activity, and interfere with meaningful personal relationships.
- Physical limitations can result in frustration, sadness, depression, and a strong sense of loss. You may miss the things you are no longer able to do.
- You may be forced to take numerous days off from work and be unable to function both at home and at the office, which may affect your employment success and family life.
- Chronic pain may be a regular occurrence.
- Limited energy may require replanning or canceling favorite activities or vacations.
- Activities, travel, or everyday events may be restricted.
- Regular physical activity and exercise may be a struggle.
- Your economical status may be affected if you incur large out-of-pocket or non-insurance-reimbursable expenses for drugs and treatment.
- Heavy menstrual flow may cause embarrassment and interfere with your social life.
- You might get migraine headaches that lead to hours or days in bed.
- Depression can make you afraid for no reason, and you may feel like you have no future.
- Sleep deprivation and emotional pain can interfere with even simple tasks.
- Your pain and other physical complaints may scare away your friends or cause others to dismiss you as a hypochondriac.

Making Changes

One very important part of coping with endometriosis is learning to take control over as much of your life as possible. This means taking an active part in treatment decisions and determining how all aspects of treatment can fit as comfortably as possible into your lifestyle. Keep in mind that there's a difference between taking control of your life and expecting a miracle such as your endometriosis going away forever. Yes, this miracle would be wonderful, but hoping . . . and waiting . . . for it will not help you improve your life. In fact, it might slow down your adjustment. Ignoring your symptoms (a type of denial) can also slow down your adjustment and limit your ability to cope. So instead of looking for miracles, focus on doing the best you can to help yourself. Because the physical pain of endometriosis can often be matched by tremendous emotional pain, it is important to acknowledge and seek help for both types of pain.

A diagnosis of endometriosis may seem totally negative, but some women may learn to view the experience positively if it serves as motivation for change or self-improvement. You see, people change and grow not only when things are going well but also during times of adversity. By looking at your life from a different perspective, you may be able to start weeding out those things that have not been good for you and begin introducing better ones. This will improve not only your own physical and emotional health but also the well-being of those around you.

Focus on altering your lifestyle to make things as easy as possible. It's important to make the right changes so that you can continue doing what you want to without putting too much pressure on your body. In fact, as you modify your life to reduce or avoid discomfort and conserve energy, you should gradually begin to feel better. For example, try to spread out your most taxing activities. Pace yourself. If necessary, be sure to include rest periods during the course of the day so that you can recharge your batteries. These changes should help you do many things while taking care of your physical needs. Following are some other suggestions that may prove helpful.

SET PRIORITIES

Look at yourself not as a person with unlimited strength but as one of decreased energy. Focus on the most important things you want to do, and try to spend less time on those that don't have as much significance.

Each day, make up a list of the things that need doing, and then group them into "musts," "maybes," and "possibilities." On some days, you'll be able to perform many of the tasks on the list; on other days, you may be able to do very few. During those times when your energy is limited, you'll be glad you were smart enough to accomplish the most important tasks first.

Just as you must complete certain tasks each day, you should also make it a point to do something you enjoy. Spend more time with the people and activities that support your physical and emotional well-being. This includes your family and others who truly care about you as a person. If you find it hard to talk to your family, choose a teacher, pastor, or a friend whom you can trust. Spend less time—or, possibly, no time!—with those people and activities that drain your strength and give you less pleasure. This will improve the overall quality of your life and equip you to deal with the stress of endometriosis.

Despite all the changes you make to better cope with your endometriosis, you must maintain as much normalcy in your life as possible. Continue doing some of the things that you enjoy the most. Don't make too many changes, because if you do, you may lose track of what your life is really all about. Hobbies can help—after all, you need something to take your mind off this disease. Find an outlet for your emotions—music, writing, photography, movies, reading, the Internet, and so on.

As you work on adapting your lifestyle, also try to modify your standards, requirements, and obligations. Don't feel that you have to meet to all of your previous standards—especially if endometriosis or its treatment has diminished your strength. Be flexible and realistic, and change as necessary to make yourself more comfortable.

Life with endometriosis has its ups and downs. Changes may be necessary because of your emotional needs, a treatment regimen, your pain, other symptoms, and a number of additional factors. The most efficient way to adjust is to anticipate as many of the ups and downs as possible and ride them out as smoothly as you can.

SET GOALS

Life without goals is meaningless. Set short-term, intermediate, and long-term goals for yourself. For instance, you might choose the next book you'd like to read, find a new hobby or interest you'd like to pursue, or plan your next vacation. Then keep moving towards these goals. This will put everything in your life into proper perspective.

LIVE LIFE ONE DAY AT A TIME

Live each day one at a time. Although this may seem incompatible with having goals, it's not. You can continue to focus on one day at a time even though you have specific goals. Enjoy life as much as you can. Try to add pleasure to some of the ordinary, mundane things in your life. If you go for a ride in your car, for example, instead of focusing on your destination, enjoy the process of getting there. Look at the scenery around you. Admire the beautiful things that life has to offer. At the same time, don't neglect planning for the future. While pain may limit some activity today, you may find a treatment that provides pain relief in the near future.

What are some of the things that you can do to improve your positive attitude? Well, a great start is to be nice to yourself. You could:

- Read a book of poetry.
- Keep in touch with old friends.
- Call your mom, dad, sister, brother, or someone else that you love.
- Don't blame yourself for mistakes.
- Spend some quality time alone.
- Read a good book—one you know and will enjoy.
- Listen to your favorite music.
- Create harmony, tranquility, and a loving atmosphere in your home.
- Put up a feeder and then sit and watch the birds.
- Watch the sun set on a warm evening.
- Take a leisurely walk and enjoy the scenery.
- Spend an afternoon at an art gallery.
- Once a year, go somewhere you've never been before.

- Respect yourself, respect others, and take responsibility for your actions.
- Go bowling, play a round of golf, or enjoy some other sport.
- Sit beside a stream, lake, fountain, or the ocean and let sound of the water soothe you.
- Dare to dream.
- Never lose sight of your goals.
- Hug your partner, your children, or your pet.
- Remember that great love and great achievements involve great risks.
- Don't let a little dispute injure a great friendship.
- Never go to bed angry.
- Open your arms to change but don't let go of your values.
- Live a good, honorable life, so when you get older and think back you will enjoy it a second time.
- Pray—there is immeasurable power in it.
- Have a lovely cup of tea.
- Pamper yourself as often as you can with a facial, manicure, or pedicure.

Getting Used to Changes

What are some of the factors that will determine how well you'll adapt to the changes in your lifestyle? There are many. For example, what were you doing before you were diagnosed with endometriosis? How satisfied were you with your work and leisure activities? How supportive were the people close to you—both family and friends? How has your condition affected you, both physically and emotionally? These and other factors will play a role in determining how you'll adjust to endometriosis, its treatment, and any changes it necessitates. But that doesn't mean your hands are tied. You can improve the way you deal with virtually any factor.

At this point, your head may be spinning. You may fear that changes will have to take place in your activity schedule, work, school, or social life. You may also be apprehensive about dealing with physical discomfort and medication. You may even worry that you won't be able to perform your normal chores and responsibilities. These concerns are in no way unusual. Many women with endometriosis feel this way. But the fact that you can do much to improve your life should help you reduce your fears and approach change in a more positive way.

As you modify your lifestyle, be aware that the changes you make can affect your self-esteem. Your self-esteem is, at least to some degree, a reflection of the role you play in life: the ways you deal with the people around you, the activities in which you're involved, and the routine you normally follow. When any of these things change, your self-esteem can change as well. By keeping this in mind, you may be more likely to make changes that will help you preserve—or improve!—your self-esteem.

What happens if you decide not to make necessary lifestyle changes? This may indicate that you're trying to deny your situation. As we discussed earlier in the book, denial is a very common coping strategy and can sometimes be positive. But it's important to be aware of its negative side as well. What if denial keeps you from doing what you need to do? For example, what if you don't get enough rest, you don't eat properly, or you don't follow your treatment regimen? This is destructive denial, and it can hurt you. Hopefully, the fact that you're reading this book in the first place shows that you're not really denying your condition. But continue to stay on top of this.

Ingredients for Successful Coping with Changes in Lifestyle

You'll be in the best shape to adapt successfully to changes in lifestyle if you:

- Understand what makes you tense, knowing what you can and cannot do to change or avoid the symptoms and problems associated with endometriosis.
- Pay attention to yourself, your aspirations and needs.
- Elicit the help of the people around you. Use relationships as a buffer. Join together with others to tackle the cause of your stress.
- Use laughter and humor to reduce stress.

- Concentrate on strengths and accomplishments rather than dwelling on negative thoughts.
- Follow a healthy diet. Eat well, especially foods high in vitamin B complex and vitamin C, to help you manage stress better. Avoid beverages with caffeine, because too much caffeine causes nervousness, irritability, and problems with digestion and sleep.
- Get enough sleep. Allow time for rest and quiet and don't try to solve problems at night or when tired.
- Exercise to reduce the effects of stress by bringing blood to the muscles and the brain and stimulate production of the chemicals that give you a sense of well-being.
- Have fun in life and have hobbies that you enjoy.
- Realize that you need to do things for yourself and actively think of yourself and not just the pain, fatigue, and other problems of this disease.
- Give yourself an identity as a beautiful person and not some tired, miserable, suffering person.
- Learn all you can about endometriosis and seek out appropriate professional help. It is important to recognize when to ask for help—medical, counseling, spiritual—whatever it takes.
- Work on enhancing your relationship with your partner, friends, and family.
- Relax to reduce your experience of pain.
- Have your mind, body, and spirit in the best shape possible, so you can constructively respond to anything that comes along.

Guidelines for Change

There are a number of things you can do to make any changes necessitated by your condition easier and less stressful. There are some general guidelines for successful living with endometriosis.

What's the best way to make lifestyle changes? Always remember that you are the most important ingredient in the recipe for successful adjustment. So do everything you can to help yourself. All of your efforts are sure to reap invaluable benefits in the form of greater health and happier day-to-day living.

- Make your house user-friendly. Every bit of energy you conserve by making things easier for yourself around the house—including the use of appliances, structural changes, clothing modifications, and more—can be funneled into areas that will better enhance your overall lifestyle.

- If you anticipate that your mobility will be limited, even temporarily, obtain a temporary handicapped parking permit from your town. In most cases you'll need a letter from your doctor saying that this is necessary. It may take time to get this permit; act now so it will be available when you need it.

- Make resting more comfortable by using support and positioning aids, made of foam, visco-elastic, or some other material. Some women use magnetic field therapy, which involves external application of an electromagnetic field to promote a sense of well being. Mattress pads, pillows, wraps, and other forms of these products provide cushioning, comfort, and support. They're light enough to be moved around the house as necessary or to take with you when you travel.

- Build up a supply of loose-fitting tops or blouses, sweatsuits, and comfortable clothing that is nonbinding and easy to put on and remove.

- Consider getting a cordless phone if you're going to be alone for any period of time. This will enable you to always have a phone close to you.

- Be aware of how your body feels—how it reacts to different activities. Then act accordingly, resting as necessary.

- Build on the talents and activities you can still enjoy—and there are sure to be plenty of them! Try to focus on the things you still have, rather than what you have lost. This guideline can be applied to relationships, activities, abilities, and interests.

- Give yourself permission to indulge in the things you enjoy. There are probably enough negative things in your life right now! Allow yourself to enjoy the positive things without guilt. A facial or a massage can do wonders for your outlook.

- Pamper yourself a little, and learn that you don't have to do everything yourself. Accept help from others when necessary, and don't overextend yourself. Have someone you love give you a relaxing massage with essential oils that are known to relax and reduce stress.
- Simplify your life. Work to reduce the pressures you place on yourself by focusing on the tasks that must be done and temporarily shelving those that are less urgent.
- Be more protective of yourself. Establish and follow routines that will supply you with the proper amounts of sleep, exercise, and nutrition. Take the precautions necessary to guard against accidents and infections.
- Improve your ability to communicate. Communication problems are the main reason relationships dissolve. By learning how to best discuss important issues, you will not only decrease the chance that your existing relationships will fail but you'll also increase the likelihood of establishing new, more enjoyable ones.
- Maintain control over your life, and do as much as you can—without exhausting yourself, of course. Research has suggested that people who continue as many of their normal routines and activities as possible feel better and recover from surgery or other procedures faster.

As We Move On

Yes, you may have to make some changes in your lifestyle. But why assume that all of them will be negative? Isn't it possible that some of them will be for the better? Maybe you've been such a hard worker that you've never spent enough time with your family. If you have to cut back on your work schedule because of endometriosis, perhaps you'll truly enjoy the increased time you'll be able to spend with your partner or children. Certainly, learning to take better care of yourself will pay off in the long run. So, as you modify your lifestyle, be sure to look for the positive.

In the remaining chapters of part III, we'll look at ways to better cope with pain, fatigue, and other effects of endometriosis and its treatment. We'll also look at diet, exercise, and medication—in other words, at many of your lifestyle concerns. So read on, and let's get your act together!

CHAPTER TWELVE

Pain

When most women think about endometriosis, it is likely that they think about pain. Pain—especially uncontrollable and intolerable pain—is probably one of the most frightening aspects of this disease.

What does the pain of endometriosis feel like? Here are some descriptions from women who have it:

- You feel so awful that you want to die so the pain will stop.
- You want to curl up into a ball and float away into space.
- Your middle feels like a truck ran over you.
- It feels like a big strong person is squeezing your intestines like a sponge.
- It feels like a sharp, stabbing pain in your side or abdomen, like a knife is cutting you while you are awake.
- The pain is so severe you become nauseated and feel faint.
- When you have sexual intercourse, it feels like your insides are being stabbed with a knife.
- Pain with sex is so bad that you dread going to bed.
- Your head pounds as if someone is beating it like a drum.
- Sharp, shooting pains run through your abdomen or your groin.

- When you urinate you get bladder spasms or sharp, stabbing pains.
- The pain is so bad that you think you will go out of your mind.
- Your lower back hurts and it is extremely sensitive to pressure of any kind.
- The pain in your back or abdomen is so strong that you can't find a comfortable position when sitting or lying down for more than a few minutes.
- The pain is so severe that the only thing that alleviates it is kneeling on the floor with your arms on a chair and rocking to and fro while puffing deep breaths.
- It feels like a burning sensation just below the pubic hairline. It feels hot and prickling, as if your insides are sitting on thorns.
- You get a knifelike pain right through the rectum, without warning. You double over, trying not to lose consciousness or black out. It gives you a raw feeling inside.
- The pain is so bad that you spend two days in bed every month during your menstrual period.
- It is tormenting. The pain is so intense that it makes you feel depressed and irritable.
- You experience mood swings and feel anxious, angry, negative.
- You feel helpless. You feel fearful and powerless.
- You worry, are insecure, and can even feel hopeless.
- The pain is so intense that you cannot imagine your life without it.
- The pain absolutely disrupts your life and at times makes it impossible to function as a normal person.
- It is pain that is the equivalent of labor and childbirth on a daily basis.

This list is not intended to frighten you but rather to show the range of feelings that women with endometriosis experience. You may have recognized yourself somewhere in one or more of those descriptions. Or, you may be thinking, "That's just not me." The amount of pain you may feel now or in the future is not necessarily related to the extent, size, or number of your endometrial growths. However, while most women with endometriosis experience pain, you might not experience it to the degree that you fear. In addition, the pain may vary and be less intense at certain times and more intense at other times. It's also very possible that much of the pain you do experience can be controlled. Once the specific type, location, and degree of pain is diagnosed, medications, surgery, or other interventions may reduce it, keep it under control, or even prevent its recurrence.

Chronic pain can be a devastating experience. Chronic pain is defined as pain that occurs, continually or intermittently, for more than six months. This usually signals an ongoing problem that cannot be eliminated through treatment. And while we know that there is no known cure for endometriosis, the pain definitely must be evaluated by a professional. Only then will you know all the options for keeping it under control so you can live your life to its fullest.

Experiencing pain can make you very fearful. Each sensation of pain may make you fear that your condition is not responding to treatment or that additional problems may be developing. And even when you are not in pain, you may fear that it's still to come. Pain also produces anxiety; this intensifies the pain and can lead to feelings of depression and helplessness. Chronic pain can also weaken the body, leaving you vulnerable to further health problems. For these reasons, pain control is a very important part of living with endometriosis. By controlling it as best you can, you will strengthen your body and enhance your well-being.

To successfully cope with pain, it's first necessary to identify its cause. Once this is done, your doctor or other healthcare professional can recommend appropriate treatments. Unfortunately, with endometriosis, it may sometimes be impossible to do anything about the underlying cause. In these instances, the pain itself, rather than the cause of the pain, is the most important concern. So if you suffer from chronic pain, it is important to find a pain management specialist who can fine-tune your medication regime or give you an opportunity to try new treatment modalities that may give you relief.

Let's learn more about pain—why it occurs with endometriosis and what treatments can be effective in controlling it.

When and Why Does Pain Occur?

Pain is a message sent from your body to your brain saying that something is wrong. This signal begins when tissue is damaged or hurt. An electrical impulse is sent through the spinal cord to the sensory center of the brain, called the *thalamus.* The signal then goes to the brain's outer layer, or *cortex.* Once the message is received in the cortex, you're able to determine the location of the pain and its intensity. Signals are then sent from the brain back through the spinal cord, triggering the release of natural painkillers such as *endorphins*—the body's own "morphine." This often diminishes the pain.

Women with endometriosis most often experience pain before and during their menstrual periods. This is usually worse than so-called normal menstrual cramps. Pain can also occur during or after sexual activity. Painful bowel movements and lower back pain just before or during menstrual periods are also very common. The Endometriosis Association reports that 96% of women with endometriosis experience pain: 95% at the time of the menstrual period; 83% at time of ovulation; and 75% at other times as well. Women also reported lower back pain, rectal and bladder pain, and migraines both before, during, and after their menstrual periods.

There are a number of reasons why women with endometriosis experience pain. For instance:

- Endometrial implants may be located right next to a nerve ending.
- Leaking endometrial lesions release inflammatory substances that can cause pain.
- Endometrial implants may compress other abdominal organs (such as the bowel, ureters, or bladder).
- Compressed endometrial nodules may be located deep in the pelvis (in areas such as the cul-de-sac).
- Endometriosis may invade the urinary tract (including the bladder or the ureters).
- Endometriosis may invade the gastrointestinal tract (the large or small intestine).
- Biochemically active endometrial lesions may secrete irritating immune system substances.
- Cysts may block blood vessels, reducing blood circulation.
- Ovarian cysts can rupture and cause intense pelvic pain or, in rare cases, peritonitis (a life-threatening infection in the lining of the abdominal and pelvic cavities).

- Lesions become engorged during the menstrual period and may cause severe menstrual cramps in the abdomen or lower back.
- Endometrial growths behind the uterus in the cul-de-sac can push the uterus into a tilted-back position, which results in pain with sex. Endometriosis on uterosacral ligaments can also cause pain with sex.
- Lesions in the area between the uterus and the rectum can cause rectal pressure and pain with bowel movements, bloating, or other intestinal upset.
- Inactivity caused by endometriosis or its treatment may lead to stiffness in your muscles or joints.
- Discomfort may occur at the site of administration of intramuscular injections.
- Endometriosis may compress or stretch pain receptors, especially when the tissues expand rapidly, as during menstruation.
- Adhesions (bands of scar tissue) bind together surfaces and vital organs, causing inflammation and chronic pain.
- Invading endometrial tissue damages vital organs.
- Malfunction of the immune system makes pain receptors more sensitive or interferes with the coding of pain signals.

There may even be reasons not yet identified. If pain is severe and not relieved, you should first call the physician who is treating you for endometriosis. In some cases, you may need to go to an emergency department or urgent care center for evaluation, because acute pain may be caused by a ruptured cyst, intestinal or ureteral obstruction (blockage of the colon or a ureter), or peritonitis following the rupture of an ovarian cyst. These are serious events. If you experience dizziness, fainting, loss of consciousness, very heavy bleeding, sustained fever, inability to pass urine, or protracted vomiting, you should seek immediate medical assessment. Acute pelvic pain may also be a symptom of pelvic inflammatory disease, appendicitis, ectopic (tubal) pregnancy, colitis, or enteritis (inflammation of the intestine). It is possible to have one of these conditions as well as endometriosis at the same time. Do not hesitate to seek medical advice if you are concerned. You should be aware, however, that many emergency department physicians are not familiar with endometriosis and the potential complications. So if you end up in this situation, always insist that your own physician, who knows your history, be contacted.

Although pain may initially be physical, your emotions can quickly worsen any pain you perceive. Anxiety or boredom, for example, can cause pain to appear more pronounced. Stress can cause muscles to tense, also increasing the degree of pain. Depression, too, may cause you to feel more pain. And, of course, pain may increase the degree to which you experience anxiety, stress, or depression, which, in turn, can lead to more pain, creating a vicious cycle.

Other factors, too, may exacerbate pain. For instance, fatigue may worsen pain by preventing your tissues from getting the rest they need to repair themselves. Your perception of pain may also vary, depending on your own tolerance as well as the degree to which you think the pain can be controlled. So, you see, the experience of pain is highly subjective, and is affected by many factors. You'll want to try to control some or all of these factors in order to manage your pain more successfully.

TREATMENT FOR PAIN

How can you start to deal with pain? One of the most important steps you can take is to use a diary and record when you feel the pain, where you feel it, how often it occurs, how long it lasts, and how intense it is. This will help you decide if the pain is something you can handle yourself or if it's serious enough to call your doctor.

Next, provide your doctor or healthcare professional with an accurate description of the pain. Describe exactly when you feel it (for example, one day before your menstrual period, for two days during your period, during ovulation, during sexual activities, etc.). Explain the exact location (for example, in your uterus, your bowel, your bladder, your rectum, your lower right side, etc.). Indicate how long you've had the pain and how long it usually lasts. Note whether the sensation is steady, sharp, throbbing, or dull. Also describe the intensity of the pain—mild, moderate, or severe. You can rate your pain using a scale that will help your doctor to understand what you are experiencing and treat you appropriately. One example of such a scale is the Mankoski Pain scale, which can help you to clearly define your individual level of pain.

Mankoski Pain Scale

0. Pain-free.
1. Very minor annoyance—occasional minor twinges. No medication needed.
2. Minor annoyance—occasional strong twinges. No medication needed.
3. Annoying enough to be distracting. Mild painkillers (e.g. aspirin, ibuprofen) take care of it.
4. Can be ignored if you are really involved in your work, but still distracting. Mild painkillers remove pain for three to four hours.
5. Can't be ignored for more than 30 minutes. Mild painkillers ameliorate pain for three to four hours.
6. Can't be ignored for any length of time, but you can still go to work and participate in social activities. Stronger painkillers (e.g. codeine, narcotics) reduce pain for three to four hours.
7. Makes it difficult to concentrate; interferes with sleep. You can still function, with effort. Stronger painkillers are only partially effective.
8. Physical activity severely limited. You can read and converse only with effort. Nausea and dizziness set in as factors of pain.
9. Unable to speak; crying out or moaning uncontrollably; near delirium.
10. Unconsciousness. Pain makes you pass out.

Remember that healthcare professionals have no way of knowing how severe your pain is unless you tell them, so don't be afraid to let them know exactly how you feel.

Identify anything that seems to relieve the pain, as well as any other symptoms that accompany the pain (for example, dizziness, nausea, fainting, heavy bleeding, inability to pass urine, diarrhea, vomiting). You should also make your doctor aware of any types of treatments you have already tried for pain relief and if they have been successful. Be sure to include both prescription and over-the-counter drugs, topical applications, herbs, acupuncture, and any other therapeutic modalities.

Why is it so important for your doctor or other healthcare professional to understand the nature of the pain you're experiencing? Only by knowing all the facts will he be able to determine the type of medication or other technique that is most appropriate in your case. You'll want to use a medication or elect to undergo a surgical procedure that will be the best way to relieve the type of pain you're experiencing.

Now, let's look at the four general categories of treatment used to control endometriosis pain: medications; surgery; physical modalities; and psychological strategies. Hormonal medications and surgery work by reducing or removing the lesions. Pain medications, physical modalities, and psychological strategies work by interrupting the transmission of pain messages before the brain receives and interprets them.

MEDICAL TREATMENT

Your doctor will recommend treatment based on the nature and location of the pain and, of course, partly on your previous responses to pain-control techniques. In the case of mild pain, aspirin and other drugs (such as nonsteroidal anti-inflammatory agents) may prove helpful. When pain is more severe, however, stronger drugs (such as narcotics) may be prescribed to decrease or eliminate the pain. Some women and physicians fear that using or prescribing narcotics will lead to drug dependence or addiction. Women with endometriosis generally experience the worst pain around the time of their menstrual periods, so they may only need strong painkillers for one or two days. In such a case the risk of addiction is quite low. (For detailed information on medications, including medications for pain, see chapter 13.)

When using medication to control the pain of endometriosis—or to control any pain—it's wise to remember that these drugs work by blocking pain signals. However, you don't want the medication to block messages that would tell you about other problems. And some drugs do have side effects you should know about. The most common ones are lightheadedness, dizziness, sedation, skin rash, nausea, vomiting, and constipation.

Sometimes medication fails to eliminate all the pain or bring it under control. In these cases, surgery may be indicated or physical modalities and psychological strategies may help.

SURGERY

Surgery may be helpful in treating the chronic pain of endometriosis when other treatment options fail or are contraindicated. In many cases, surgery for endometriosis turns out to be the best route to pain relief. Fortunately, even a relatively minor surgery can bring great relief.

We've discussed surgical procedures in chapter 2. For pain, the most common surgical approach is a laparoscopy. Using this procedure, a doctor skilled in treating endometriosis can diagnose the problem, identify where endometrial growths are located, determine which vital organs are involved, and remove endometrial lesions and adhesions. A laparotomy is more invasive but may be necessary in some cases. Videolaseroscopy is used to remove endometrial lesions, cysts, and other problems that can cause chronic pain. A new procedure, pain mapping, uses a microlaparoscope and allows a doctor to touch the woman's abdominal organs to locate specific areas that are painful. For many women, these surgical procedures can result in a significant alleviation of symptoms.

For those who are severely incapacitated by endometriosis pain, radical surgery may be a consideration. This usually involves a total hysterectomy—removal of the uterus and both ovaries and excision of adhesions, endometrial lesions, and cysts. Even as a last resort, however, this radical procedure does not always eliminate endometriosis completely.

Regardless of what type of surgery you are considering, it is absolutely imperative that you find a top-notch endometriosis specialist. A good surgeon will thoroughly examine and attempt to remove all traces of endometriosis, even when it is located in hard-to-reach areas. If you have radical surgery, you need a skilled surgeon to recognize and remove the endometriosis, place sutures appropriately, and complete a repair that will minimize the pain that may occur with sex. Whether you have surgery or decide against it, it is important to find a healthcare professional who will work with you to provide holistic and comprehensive care.

For more details on these surgeries refer to chapter 2.

PHYSICAL MODALITIES

The localized pain of endometriosis can often be effectively relieved with one or more types of physical modalities such as heat, cold, massage, energy medicine, acupuncture, and magnetic field therapy. By pinpointing the location, frequency, and intensity of the pain, a knowledgeable healthcare professional can determine which type of physical modality is most likely to help your specific circumstances.

Heat

Heat can be a very beneficial way of relaxing and soothing your muscles to relieve soreness and pain. This is called thermotherapy. It's considered to be the oldest form of pain reliever, or analgesic. If you are going to use heat, be careful about how intense it is and how long you apply it. Too much heat for too long a period of time is not advisable. Don't assume that if a little bit of heat is good, a lot of heat can be better. This is a good way to get burned!

Some professionals recommend applying heat with a hot water bottle, an electric heating pad, a microwaveable gel pad, or a wet towel. Hot baths or showers may also be helpful. Just be sure to take any precautions necessary to avoid burns. For instance, do not use a heating pad on high for a long period of time, and do not allow yourself to fall asleep while using any type of heating pad.

Cold

Although there are many benefits to using heat, some women with endometriosis respond better to cold treatment. Cold often can be even more effective than heat, providing faster and longer-lasting relief. Cold treatment, also known as cryotherapy, can help by numbing the nerve endings in the affected areas. It also decreases the activity of the cells.

One common method of cold treatment involves soaking a cloth or towel in ice water, wringing it out, and applying it to the painful area. Gel packs, which can be obtained from pharmacies and medical supply stores, are an excellent means of applying cold and, because of their pliable consistency, are often more comfortable than ice packs. These gel packs are kept in the freezer, removed for use, and then refrozen. Of course, if you don't have a gel pack, ice cubes or a frozen wet cloth placed in a plastic bag can be just as effective. As with hot compresses, be sure to wrap these applications in a towel before holding it against the skin. And make sure you follow professional recommendations regarding how to use any of these techniques or procedures.

Some women don't like cold treatments, saying that they're only good for polar bears. Others, however, find that they provide greater pain relief than heat treatments.

Massage

Massage is another useful physical modality for reducing pain. For centuries, the therapeutic use of touch has been applied to heal the body and reduce stress and tension. Practitioners often use a combination of bodywork techniques (such as acupressure, reflexology, polarity therapy, and therapeutic touch) to help balance energy in the body and bring about enhanced well-being. Prolonged tension can often cause pain. Massage helps to release tension and promote relaxation; it also helps break up the waste deposits concentrated in muscles and other tissues and stimulates circulation.

Massage can be performed by a professional or a partner or you can perform it yourself, provided that the uncomfortable area is accessible to you and you can use the technique effectively. To maximize both safety and effectiveness, be sure to check with a physician, physical therapist, or massage professional before attempting to use massage as a means of controlling your pain.

Energy Medicine Devices

Energy (or bioenergetic) medicine refers to therapies that use an energy field—electrical, magnetic, sonic, acoustic, microwave, or infrared—to treat health conditions. Energy medicine uses diagnostic screening devices to measure the various electromagnetic frequencies emitted by the body to detect imbalances in the body's energy fields and then correct them. Most energy medicine devices are based on the acupuncture meridian system (the network of energy channels throughout the body). Examples of commonly used treatment devices are the TENS unit (explained below); a type of device that uses a lower electrical current than the TENS unit and radiates photons of light to help restore the cell's normal energy state; and an instrument that uses radio waves to produce short, intense electromagnetic pulses that can penetrate deep into the tissues of the body.

TENS Units. TENS stands for *transcutaneous electrical nerve stimulation*. These devices are widely used in doctors' offices and physiotherapy clinics, and can be used at home. The TENS unit is a little box about the size of a cigarette pack. It contains a generator that has wire leads with electrodes at the ends of them. The unit may have anywhere from 2 to 40 electrode wire leads. A little gel is attached to the electrodes, and then they're placed on your skin, on or near the area to be treated. When you turn on the unit, a low level of electricity flows into the area from the TENS unit. This stimulates the nerve fibers and blocks the transmission of pain messages to the brain. Shocking, right? Don't worry. You probably won't even feel anything, or you may just experience a mild tingling sensation.

One of the problems with TENS units is that their effectiveness seems to decrease as time goes by. Efficacy also seems to be related to your diligence, the knowledge of your therapist, and the appropriate placing of electrodes.

If you want to get a TENS unit, you usually need a prescription from your physician. A nurse or physical therapist will then teach you how to place the electrodes to provide maximum pain relief. But it's probably a good idea to rent a machine before buying one to see if it works for you.

Acupuncture

Another pain relief technique—one that has gained increasing acceptance by professionals in the last few years—is *acupuncture*. This ancient Chinese technique is based on the belief that health is determined by a balanced flow of *chi* (also known as *qi*), the vital energy present in all living organisms. An acupuncturist inserts very thin needles at various depths and angles at specific points predetermined to bring about pain relief. The needles suppress pain perception and may also trigger the release of endorphins and enkephalins, the body's natural painkilling chemicals. In fact, in China, acupuncture is often used as an anesthetic during surgery, indicating a high degree of effectiveness in many cases.

Although the insertion of needles may sound painful, patients rarely experience anything more than occasional, temporary discomfort. If you are interested in trying acupuncture, speak to your physician or other healthcare professional, who should be able to refer you to a qualified professional.

Magnetic Field Therapy

Recently, scientists have discovered that external magnetic fields can affect the body's functioning. The healing effect of magnets is possible because the body's nervous system is governed in part by varying patterns of currents and electromagnetic fields. Magnetic fields can stimulate metabolism and increase the amount of oxygen available to cells.

Magnetic therapy is applied in many ways and may be used to alleviate pain and other symptoms. Treatment times and duration vary. To better understand the therapeutic use of magnets, consult a practitioner for guidance.

TRADITIONAL CHINESE MEDICINE

Traditional Chinese medicine (TCM) is an ancient method of health care that combines the use of medicinal herbs (see chapter 15 for more detailed information about herbs), acupuncture, nutrition, massage, and therapeutic exercise. An approach to health and healing that is very different from traditional or modern Western medicine, TCM looks for the underlying causes of imbalances in the body. It focuses more on the response of the patient to the disease than on the disease itself. This approach is well suited to the woman who wants to assume more responsibility for her own healing.

HERBAL REMEDIES AND DIETARY SUPPLEMENTS

Herbs and certain dietary supplements can be effective when used over an extended period of time to help reduce bloating, cramping, and pain. For women with endometriosis, they can be excellent secondary therapeutic agents to help with pain relief. For example, the herb vitex has been shown to help reestablish the normal balance of estrogen and progesterone during a woman's menstrual cycle. It stimulates the pituitary gland to produce more luteinizing hormone, which leads to a greater production of progesterone. Dong quai (an herb used in traditional Chinese medicine) also helps to promote normal hormone balance.

Many women find that certain dietary supplements lessen endometriosis pain. One of these is evening primrose oil. It contains gamma linolenic acid (GLA), a fatty acid the body converts to a hormonelike substance that has antiinflammatory properties.

Vitamins and minerals also play a role in pain relief. Vitamin C with bioflavonoids, vitamin E, and B complex vitamins (B1, B6, and B12) and minerals, including zinc and magnesium, may help to reduce pain and inflammation of endometriosis. However, you should only take herbs and nutritional supplements, vitamins, or minerals under the supervision of a nutritionally oriented doctor. You can read more about these and other important dietary considerations in chapter 15.

As you can see, there are several physical modalities that can be used for pain relief, most of which can be used at home. These can be helpful by themselves or in combination with medication, surgery, other alternative therapies, or psychological strategies. You can further enhance the effectiveness of these techniques by being sure to get the proper balance of rest and exercise. (See chapters 14 and 16 for details on how rest and exercise can help you better cope with endometriosis.)

PSYCHOLOGICAL STRATEGIES

As we discussed earlier in this chapter, there are many factors that may influence how you experience pain, such as anxiety, depression, and stress. Once you learn to control these factors, you're sure to feel a lot better. This is not to say that the pain is "all in your head." But pain is usually a combination of physiological and psychological factors. So although you may be experiencing true physiological pain, your mind is very much involved in determining exactly how much it hurts.

What does all this mean? If medication, surgery, alternative therapies, and various physical modalities don't alleviate your pain, you can still relieve some—if not all—of it by working on your mind's *perception* of the pain. Many people have found effective pain control through the use of relaxation techniques, imagery, hypnotherapy, and biofeedback. These techniques work by separating you from your sensations of pain, enabling you to feel better. It is easy to learn some of them at home. Others must be taught by professionals. The following discussions should help you decide which of the psychological pain control techniques may best help you as you learn to cope with pain caused by the effects of endometriosis.

Relaxation Techniques

You know now that tension can actually increase your pain. So it makes sense that relaxation—the opposite of tension—can help you reduce your overall level of pain. As an added benefit, using relaxation techniques may increase your general sense of well-being and help you deal better with the stress of many day-to-day problems—not just those related to endometriosis.

In chapter 9, you learned how imagery may be used to induce relaxation. Other procedures include progressive relaxation, meditation, autogenics, deep breathing, and a method called the Quick Release. Let's look briefly at each of these techniques.

Progressive relaxation is based on the premise that when you experience anything stressful, the body responds with muscle tension—which, of course, can increase pain. In this procedure, which is usually performed for 15 to 20 minutes once or twice daily, you sequentially tense and then relax the different muscle groups in your body, one group at a time. If you wish to learn more about this popular and effective technique, don't hesitate to consult books at your local library or speak to a professional.

Meditation is a valuable tool for stress reduction. It really is a name for any activity that keeps the attention calmly anchored in the present moment. When the mind is quiet and focused in the present, it is neither reacting to memories from the past nor preoccupied with plans for the future, two major sources of stress. Meditation can allow you to achieve a deep level of relaxation in a short period of time. During meditation, you focus your mind, uncritically, on one object, sound, activity, or experience and detach from any extraneous thoughts. Depending on the type of meditation you choose to use, this technique usually works best when taught by a professional or learned from a reliable book or videotape.

Autogenics is a systematic program that helps you train your body and mind to respond to your own verbal commands to relax. With this procedure, which can be used for short periods of time and repeated as frequently as needed, you give yourself verbal suggestions of heaviness, warmth, and calmness. Again, a book on relaxation techniques or a qualified professional can guide you in the use of this procedure.

Many people find that *deep breathing* can significantly increase their relaxation and, as a result, decrease their pain. Deep breathing can be used in a number of different ways. Here's one simple deep-breathing exercise. First, assume a comfortable position on your bed or on the floor. Then put one hand on your abdomen and the other on your chest. Inhale slowly and deeply through your nose, so that the hand on your abdomen moves higher. Hold your breath as long as you're comfortable doing so; then exhale slowly through your mouth, making a peaceful "whooshing" sound. Feel the hand on your abdomen sink slowly, and allow a growing feeling of relaxation to deepen inside you. Repeat this sequence for five to ten minutes. Then give yourself a few minutes to become aware of your surroundings before getting up. Practice this technique at least twice a day, extending its length if you wish.

Another simple but effective relaxation technique is the *Quick Release.* Close your eyes, take a deep breath, and hold it as you tighten the muscles in every part of your body that you can think of—your fists, arms, legs, stomach, neck, buttocks, and so on. Continue to hold your breath and to keep your muscles tense for about six seconds. Then let your breath out in a "whoosh," and allow the tension to drain out of your muscles. Let your body go limp. Keep your eyes closed, and breathe rhythmically and comfortably for about 20 seconds. Repeat this tension-relaxation cycle three times. By the end of the third repetition, you'll probably feel a lot more relaxed. Keep on practicing this technique, as continuous practice will condition your body to respond quickly and completely.

You may find other relaxation techniques that are helpful. Remember that your ability to increase relaxation and decrease pain by means of the mind-body connection are limited only by your imagination. Don't overlook this valuable way of improving your sense of well-being.

Imagery

Imagery is the process of conjuring up mental pictures or scenes in order to harness your body's energy. These images (that either occur spontaneously or that you guide in particular directions) are "multisensory"—you can see, hear, feel, smell, or taste them in your own mind. By using positive mental images, you may be able to more effectively cope with and reduce pain. Guided imagery often results in a positive physical response that reduces stress, slows the heart rate, and stimulates the immune system. The technique can be used to control headaches, hypertension, depression, and pain. Sometimes used alone, imagery can also be used in combination with prescribed medical treatment.

How can you use imagery to control the pain of endometriosis? Get into a relaxed position in a comfortable chair or in bed. The lights should be dimmed, and outside sounds or noises should be minimized. Try to avoid interruptions. Breathe smoothly and rhythmically, allowing your body to release tension and relax. Then imagine a scene of your own choosing, trying to make the image as vivid and real as possible. This scene can be used therapeutically to help you feel better, as the following example demonstrates.

Ann was experiencing a sharp pain in her abdomen and worked with an expert in applying imagery procedures to get some relief. She was instructed to relax and then develop an image of what this pain looked like. She imagined it as dozens of very sharp pins being jabbed into the area. She was then instructed to slowly reverse the action she had pictured. So Ann imagined the pins slowly being removed from her abdomen and a soothing, healing cream being applied. Finally, the pins were completely out. Ann was then able to deepen her relaxation, greatly reducing her discomfort.

There are other images you can use to reduce pain. For example, you could initially imagine your insides being hit by a hammer or tightly squeezed by a woodshop vise. Then, to reverse the image, you could imagine the hammer being removed or the vise being loosened. Or you might think of cool air being blown across the affected area or of the area being surrounded by warm water in a bathtub. Imagery is restricted only by your creativity, and can be used anywhere. (Have you ever taken a bath on a bus?!) Two good books on the subject are *In the Mind's Eye* by Arnold Lazarus and *Visualization for Change* by Patrick Fanning. See if your public library or local bookstore has them.

Hypnotherapy

Hypnotherapy is a calm repetition of words and statements designed to induce a state of deep relaxation in which there is a heightened receptivity to suggestion. During this state, verbal suggestions help the mind to block your awareness of pain and replace it with a more positive feeling. Many doctors combine hypnotherapy with traditional treatments. Recent studies show that 94% of patients benefit from hypnotherapy, even if the only benefit is relaxation. While hypnotherapy is often quite effective for pain control, it doesn't work for everybody. Also, in some cases, it won't help with severe pain.

You can learn how to hypnotize yourself so that you can do so whenever you need it. You must first be taught this technique by a professional—a licensed psychologist, social worker, or certified hypnotherapist, for instance. Many good books on clinical hypnosis can give you further information about this valuable tool. Organizations such as the American Institute of Hypnotherapy, the American Society of Clinical Hypnosis, the International Medical and Dental Hypnotherapy Association, or the National Guild of Hypnotists can refer you to a legitimate practitioner in your area.

Biofeedback

Biofeedback uses the techniques of relaxation and imagery, in conjunction with modern technology, to teach you how to change and control your body's vital functions. Simple electronic devices measure your response and give feedback in the form of sounds or images, letting you know what's going on inside your body. In fact, biofeedback provides moment-by-moment information about the effect that your imagery and relaxation techniques are having on your physiological responses. What do we mean by physiological responses? Skin temperature, the electrical conductivity of the skin, muscle tension, heart rate, and brain wave activity are all physiological responses that can be measured using biofeedback.

How, exactly, can biofeedback help you control pain? Electrodes connected to the biofeedback unit are taped or otherwise attached to your skin. Then you use meditation, relaxation, visualization, or some other technique to bring about the desired response. These electrodes monitor your body's response and transmit the information they pick up back to the biofeedback unit in the form of electrical impulses. The unit then translates this feedback into sounds, lights, or pictures that you can hear or observe. Using this information, you can experiment and find the types of imagery and other relaxation techniques that will allow you to best control your internal responses to reduce muscle pain.

Jenny was experiencing a lot of cramping pain, so her physician suggested that she try biofeedback. A machine measuring muscle tension was attached to the area of her body where she was experiencing the pain, in much the same way that electrodes from an EKG machine are connected. (Don't worry. There is no pain, and you won't get jolted!) As Jenny attempted to relax her muscles in that area, the machine let her know if she was really relaxing and also how well she was doing. As she became aware of her lessening tension, Jenny learned which mental images worked best for her. Eventually she was able to use the imagery on her own, without the machine, to help control her pain.

Certified biofeedback professionals can be found throughout the country. Good resources for names of local practitioners include your physician, your local hospital or clinic, and the Association for Applied Psychophysiology and Biofeedback.

Coping Strategies

By now you probably understand the connection between emotions and pain and want to do everything you can to decrease your fear, stress, tension, and other negative emotions—emotions that may make you more aware of pain or even increase it. Part II should help you pinpoint the source of your emotional distress and suggests ways to better cope with your feelings. If you haven't already read these chapters, now would be a great time to give them a try. Never underestimate the effect that emotions can have on your physical health!

Of course, the more time you have to think about your pain, the worse it will seem. So try to divert your attention. Develop interests that require concentration—computer games, crafts, crossword puzzles, or whatever suits your fancy. You can always come up with activities and thoughts that will entertain your mind while increasing feelings of physical well-being.

Pain-Control Resources

You can learn and gain access to many pain-control techniques from your own physician, from mental health professionals, including psychologists and social workers who specialize in certain pain-control techniques, and from other healthcare professionals. Or you may want to read some of the books on pain control that are available in libraries and bookstores. Certainly, many techniques can be used at home—although, in some cases, they may work better if you learn them from clinics or centers. In fact, certain clinics specialize in the control of pain.

If you decide to consult a pain management specialist, there are both diagnostic and therapeutic types. Various tests can be administered at a diagnostic center to determine more about the causes of your pain and the pathways involved. These include thermography (mapping the body's surface temperature), spinogram (measures the involvement of the spinal pathways), selected blind nerve blocks (injections to identify the nerves or nerve bundles involved in the pain), and neurological assessments. The results from these tests may help you and your doctor make decisions about surgery and medication. A therapeutic pain clinic or center will identify a combination of medication, adjunctive treatments (such as biofeedback, physiotherapy, and others), exercise programs, and group counseling that can help relieve pain, improve your general health, and strengthen coping skills. Be sure to seek out a pain management center or specialist who is up to date on the complexities of endometriosis-associated pain.

You might also want to get involved in a support group specifically for people living with pain. Examples of such organizations are the National

Chronic Pain Outreach and the American Chronic Pain Association. (See the resources section for a more complete listing.) These groups have chapters throughout the country, and more are always forming. It can be comforting to know that you're not alone in trying to cope with pain. You may even learn some new pain control strategies.

Despite the effectiveness of the many pain-control techniques available today, it's important to consult your physician to make sure that any or all of the techniques you're considering are appropriate for you and will pose no danger to your health. And, of course, your physician may make you aware of further coping techniques, one of which might be just the ticket!

Pain-Control Ideas

There are a number of additional things you can do to relieve the pain of endometriosis:

- Employ a take-charge approach to endometriosis.
- Get plenty of rest.
- Take control of your medical treatment. Become a partner with your doctor or other healthcare professional. Learn as much as you can to enable you to make the best possible decisions for yourself.
- Eat healthy foods (see chapter 15).
- Take nutritional supplements that are known to reduce inflammation.
- Evaluate the benefits and actions of certain herbs that may help. Some of the ones indicated for endometriosis pain include astragalus, garlic, goldenseal, myrrh gum, pau d'arco, and red clover, which have antibiotic and antitumor properties; and burdock root, dong quai, and red raspberry leaf, which help to balance hormones. (See chapter 15 for additional information.)
- Keep a daily pain diary. It will give you a clearer picture of your pain, and help you to anticipate it and to determine if it has a regular pattern or length of duration. You'll feel more in control if you know what to expect.

- Concentrate on having normal cycles and relaxing rather than on negative experiences.
- Be active, despite the pain.
- Maximize your use of stress-reduction techniques.
- Allow yourself to cry—it is a surprisingly helpful way of ridding the body of toxins and reducing pain.
- Do things that bring you a sense of fulfillment, joy, and purpose.
- Maintain a positive attitude. Hang up inspirational sayings. Talk to yourself in a positive manner.
- Pay close and loving attention to yourself, tuning in to all your needs.
- Release all negative emotions. Express your feelings.
- Accept yourself and everything in your life as an opportunity for growth and learning.
- When fear of, or from, pain occurs, focus on images that evoke feelings of peace or joy.
- Keep a sense of humor.
- Take care of yourself—nourishing, supporting, and encouraging yourself.
- Hold positive images and goals in your mind.

An Unagonizing Conclusion

Unfortunately, pain is the most common symptom experienced with endometriosis. But don't throw in the heating pad! Realize that the pain need not last forever. A lot can be done, both medically and psychologically, to increase your level of comfort and help you more fully enjoy each and every day.

CHAPTER THIRTEEN

Medication

Medication is one of the main interventions for managing many of the symptoms associated with endometriosis. In chapter 2 we presented the hormonal medications used to treat endometriosis. This chapter contains more detail about their potential side effects and suggestions for minimizing them. In addition to medications prescribed specifically for endometriosis, this chapter examines other drugs that can help you control anxiety, depression, and pain.

The value of medication as a treatment varies, depending on its therapeutic goal. Different medications are prescribed for different reasons. Some drugs work well to reduce the anatomic manifestations of endometriosis (in other words, shrink growths or stop new growths from occurring). Others are prescribed with the goal of reducing pain. Still others are prescribed in the hopes of improving a woman's chances of becoming pregnant. While there are medications that have been proven to shrink or stop growths and to reduce or even stop pain, there is no medication currently available that enhances fertility among women with endometriosis.

The decision to use certain medications is highly personal. Some women welcome drugs as a powerful means of controlling physical symptoms or emotional problems. Others are afraid of their power and of eventually becoming dependent on them. Still others resent the presence of any artificial substance in their bodies. Where do your feelings fit in?

Regardless of what your attitudes are about using medication, your physician may indicate that you don't have much choice in the matter. But you do! Evaluate the actions of each medication, as well as the potential benefits and side effects. Your level of pain may make drugs a more desirable option, or you may want to try medical treatment before proceeding with surgery. Taking medication is not enough, though. You must take it properly: the right drug, the right dose, at the right time, for the right length of time. Otherwise it can be ineffective—or very dangerous.

Let's talk more about medications so that, if you do choose to take them, you'll be informed and able to maximize safety and effectiveness, and minimize their potential side effects.

Choosing the Appropriate Medication

How does a doctor determine which medication has the best chance to alleviate your specific symptoms and endometriosis-related problems? In prescribing a drug program, your physician will take into consideration the severity of your endometriosis, as well as the symptoms you're experiencing; any other treatments you are using; your age; and your overall health, among other factors. If, in the past, you have shown sensitivities or allergies to any drugs, you should certainly let your healthcare professional know—even if you think this information is already part of your medical record. The more facts you relate, the better chance of finding the right treatment for you.

Your doctor cannot know how a given medication will affect you or your endometriosis. Sometimes it's necessary to alter your treatment plan. This can be frustrating, but keep in mind that the right drug—or combination of drugs—may greatly increase your comfort level. So try to be patient!

Knowing How and When to
Take Your Medication

Whenever your doctor prescribes a medication, be sure you understand exactly what the drug is supposed to do, how and when it should be taken, how long you are expected to take it, and what potential side effects you may experience. For example, certain medications should be taken only after meals, while others must be taken on an empty stomach. In still other cases, specific foods must be avoided during drug therapy. Be sure to obtain and read a copy of the package insert for each medication you take. This will explain how the drug works in the body and list indications for use, possible side effects, contraindications, and other valuable information. As we'll discuss later, your pharmacist is a good resource.

Each person has different needs as far as dosage and frequency of drugs are concerned. Even if somebody you know has the same symptoms that are troubling you and is taking the same medication, her dosage may not necessarily be appropriate for you. And once you start taking any drug, the dosage may have to be adjusted on the basis of any side effects you're experiencing and how well the medication is managing your symptoms.

Very few physicians will keep you on high doses of any medication unless they feel it's absolutely essential. Still, if you're taking a substantial amount of any drug and question the need for it, don't be afraid to discuss your concerns with a healthcare professional. If you're feeling good and would like to reduce your dosage—or to stop taking the drug altogether—by all means, speak to your doctor. Together you will be able to plan a schedule for reducing your dosage and, if possible, ending treatment.

They Might Not Get Along!

Never take any medications other than those prescribed for you without first checking with your healthcare professional. If you need to take many different drugs, it's important to avoid altering your dosage or changing the times you take the medication. Follow your doctor's prescription exactly as written.

If you see physicians other than those who are treating your endometriosis, be aware that they may prescribe medications that should not be taken with your endometriosis medications. Some mixes can make your symptoms worse, interfere with the action of endometriosis drugs, or cause additional problems. For example, if you are taking an endometriosis medication in the form of a nasal spray, you should not use a topical nasal decongestant for at least two hours after your dose. Many drugs prescribed for endometriosis result in a small loss in bone density over the course of treatment. You should not take anticonvulsants or corticosteroids with medications that result in bone density loss. Drugs you may take for endometriosis pain, such as tranquilizers, acetaminophen, or narcotics, should never be mixed with alcohol. MAO inhibitors (prescribed for depression) should not be taken with antihistamines or decongestants.

It makes sense to have one primary physician in charge of your care. Any other healthcare professional you see can then consult as necessary to verify that the treatment strategies will work together. Because certain medications are chemically incompatible, you should never mix drugs without first knowing that the combination is safe. Don't take the chance. Check it out. And always make sure that everyone treating you for the symptoms associated with endometriosis knows all the medications you're taking.

Side Effects

You should be aware of the possible side effects of any prescribed (or over-the-counter) medication. Side effects, as you know, are the less-than-pleasant effects a drug may have on your body. Hot flashes, headaches, insomnia, vaginal dryness, decreased sex drive—these are all possible adverse effects of drugs commonly prescribed for endometriosis. In addition, depression, fatigue, acne, joint pain, dizziness, increased sex drive, nausea, short-term memory loss, sweating, or significant loss of bone density can occur with some drugs.

Clearly, however, adverse effects are one of the biggest concerns about taking medication, and they may occur whenever a drug is taken. If the side effects you experience are slight, they probably won't upset you—especially if the medication you're taking is producing the desired effect. Even if the side effects are disturbing, you may want to continue the medication if potential benefits outweigh any problems you're experiencing. However, if you experience excessive discomfort, you should discuss this with your healthcare professional and weigh the disadvantages against the advantages to determine if the medication should be continued, changed, or stopped.

With any drug, the goal is to find the lowest effective dose that will maximize the therapeutic value and minimize any side effects. Again, if there are any problems, call your doctor!

WHAT CAN BE DONE?

Unpleasant, adverse effects can be minimized. Let's discuss some of the things that you can do to either minimize or better cope with some of the most common side effects of the drugs frequently prescribed for endometriosis.

Hot Flashes

Did someone just turn up the heat to 500°F? Does your chest suddenly feel warm, with the heat quickly spreading to your face and neck? If so, chances are you are experiencing a hot flash. Relax! They are temporary, and there are several remedies that can provide relief. Women find many ways to cope with hot flashes. Experiment to find what works best for you in your own particular setting. Here are some suggestions. While it might seem obvious, keep cool. Heat or sudden, dramatic temperature swings can trigger hot flashes, so try to avoid these situations. Wear layered or loose clothing made of fibers that help to disperse heat and perspiration. As soon as you feel a flash coming, loosen any tight clothing. Other tactics, like fanning yourself, splashing on cool water, turning down the heat, opening a window, or taking off your shoes, can help. Concentrate on regulating your breathing. Take nine or ten slow, deep, comfortable breaths. Repeat this for several minutes until the hot flash passes. Drink something cool. Put a dampened cloth in a plastic bag in the freezer so it's ready to take with you wherever you go. At night, take it out and put it beside your bed. Visualize yourself sitting by a lake with a cool breeze blowing. Before bed, relax in a tub of warm water until the water cools. Take plenty of showers.

Eat healthy. Following a diet high in complex carbohydrates and low in fat can help. Caffeine, alcohol, sugar, spicy foods, hot soups, hot drinks, and very large meals may trigger hot flashes because they stimulate the production of norephinephrine. So avoid them! Eat many small meals rather than three large ones. Fill up with soybean products, which contain phytoestrogens—natural plant compounds that act like estrogen. Drink lots of water and organic fruit juices. To help with night sweats, keep a carafe of ice water on your night table and sip as needed. Herbal teas and infusions can also help. An infusion is a brew of medicinal herbs. It can be made by letting the herbs sit after covering with boiling water or by setting the herbs and water in sunlight. Usually, the leaves, flowers, or other delicate parts of a plant are used in an infusion. Drink the infusion immediately upon arising and two or three times each day, as recommended by an herbalist, or consult a book on herbal healing. Various herbs, such as Siberian ginseng, dong quai, fo ti, black cohosh, and wild yam also help many women. (More information can be found in chapter 15.)

You may want to investigate homeopathic remedies, specific solutions and combination formulas that are dilutions of natural substances from plants, minerals, and animals. Homeopathic medicine matches different symptom patterns or "profiles" of illness and uses solutions that act to stimulate the body's natural healing response.

Additionally, some women find that vitamin E minimizes or eliminates both hot flashes and vaginal dryness. Natural progesterone, in skin cream or capsule form, may also provide relief.

Exercise and stress-reduction techniques will also help to alleviate hot flashes. (See chapters 9 and 16 for more information on these techniques.)

Keep talking. Break the taboos against hot flashes. Let people know when you are having a hot flash and convince yourself—and others—that it is nothing to be ashamed of. Use positive, not demeaning, humor, such as "It's not a hot flash, it's a POWER SURGE!"

Finally, keep track of your hot flashes to see if a pattern emerges. The more you know about yourself, the better you will be able to manage this problem and the better you will feel. Reducing the element of surprise will help you to take control of your body and be better prepared.

Vaginal Dryness

Insufficient lubrication during sexual activity can be very painful, but you can improve comfort by following some simple strategies. First, be sure to eliminate any irritants that may be the culprits (such as latex condoms, bubble baths, douches, contraceptive creams, laundry detergents, or spermicides). Commercial lubricants, such as Replens, Astro-Glide, or K-Y Jelly can help. In addition, cold-pressed castor oil, hydrogels, vitamin E oil or suppositories, and sesame or other high-quality oils used during sex or rubbed on delicate dry tissues can all be soothing. Vitamin E can be taken orally and also applied directly to vaginal tissue. Add moisture to your tissues by drinking eight cups of water daily. Herbs such as dandelion leaf and oat straw, taken orally, may help restore vaginal lubrication. If you are taking antibiotics, you may experience dryness due to an imbalance in pH. Try adding yogurt with active cultures to restore the natural balance.

Massaging the vagina regularly through intercourse, sexual play, or self-stimulation will help thicken the vaginal wall and alleviate painful intercourse. Having sex before you are fully lubricated can cause both irritation and pain. Prolong the cuddling, stroking, caressing, and kissing before intercourse and other foreplay to give yourself more time to get aroused and lubricated. (See chapter 22 for more information about sex.)

You can also use visualization to reverse vaginal dryness. For example, during a relaxation procedure, visualize the area as healthy, pink, moist and desirable rather than uncomfortably dry.

Avoid products that may cause or contribute to dryness, such as antihistamines, douches, sprays, and colored or perfumed toilet paper and soaps that can irritate the tissues of the vulva.

Mood or Memory Changes

Certain drugs cause hormonal shifts that can make us particularly moody. Just a few simple tricks can help you head them off at the pass. If you feel yourself slipping into depression or anxiety, act, don't brood. Get up and take a walk, play with your dog, do something you normally enjoy—something that gives you a sense of control and accomplishment. Exercise for 15 minutes to stimulate endorphins. Call a friend. Find out how other women handle mood swings. Use relaxation techniques to work off stress, anxiety, or depression.

A good diet with adequate protein is important. Eat well and listen to your body. Try foods that set off a series of chemical reactions in your brain that help invigorate you. For example, eat a snack that combines protein with carbohydrates—like half a turkey sandwich. Or try an all-carbohydrate snack like a bagel if you are free-falling into anxiety. Stop the caffeine and alcohol. Nutritional supplements such as St. John's wort, supercholine, pantothenic acid, Vitamin B complex, ginkgo leaf extract, and protein powders can help enhance both mood and memory. Other alternative therapies, including homeopathic medicine, hypnotherapy, light therapy, magnetic field therapy, and traditional Chinese medicine can also help improve mood swings and memory loss.

Bone Density Loss

Certain medications prescribed for endometriosis result in decreased levels of estrogen and progesterone. The loss of estrogen triggers an increase in bone resorption or bone loss. This reduces bone mass, which means a higher risk of fractures. Bone mass—the amount of mineral in the bone—generally reaches its peak when a woman is between the ages of 30 and 35. After that, it begins to decline. So taking certain medications prescribed for endometriosis, along with nature's own timing, can result in bone density loss. Bone thinning can also result from excessive use of alcohol or smoking. In addition, a family history of osteoporosis predisposes a woman to bone thinning either at an earlier age or at a faster rate.

It is critical to take calcium supplements (along with magnesium and vitamin D) when you are taking any endometriosis medications that may cause bone density loss and after natural or surgical menopause. Other things you can do to promote bone health include following a high–complex carbohydrate, low-fat diet. Many additional suggestions can be found in chapter 15.

Here, again, natural progesterone cream may be helpful because it is absorbed through the skin and will aid in building bone mass. Some of the other alternative therapies we have already mentioned, such as traditional Chinese medicine and homeopathic remedies, could be used. Stay, or get, active. Increase weight-bearing exercises (subject to approval from your physician) such as walking, biking or weight training . . . anything that puts weight on the bones. Above all, stop smoking.

Insomnia

Do you ever find yourself tossing and turning all night when everyone else in the house is asleep? Do you ever feel like you would do just about anything to get a good night's sleep? Then you probably are suffering from insomnia. A common cause of insomnia is night sweats (those hot flashes we mentioned earlier). If you are taking a medication that produces menopause-like symptoms, you may suffer from insomnia as a result.

Here are a few tips to help you get some shut-eye. Turn your clock to the wall. Staring at it will only make you more tense. Get out of bed if you are still awake after 20 minutes. Do something dull that will make you sleepy. Make sure that your bedroom is not too hot or too cold. Most people sleep best in a cool room, so turn down the thermostat when you turn out the lights.

Modify your diet by adding foods that can help induce sleep. For example, turkey, bananas, figs, dates, yogurt, milk, tuna, whole grain crackers, and nut butter are high in tryptophan, which promotes sleep. Avoid certain foods that contain tyramine (which increases the release of norepinephrine, a brain stimulant) before bedtime. Examples are bacon, cheese, chocolate, eggplant, ham, potatoes, sauerkraut, sugar, sausage, spinach, tomatoes, and wine. Stop drinking caffeine-containing beverages after lunch. It may help to consult a dietitian who can help you make specific adjustments to your diet and can recommend appropriate substitutions.

Avoid alcohol in the evening because it usually disrupts deep sleep cycles. Tobacco contains nicotine, a neurostimulant that can cause sleep problems, so be sure that this is not the culprit. Certain nasal decongestants and cold medications have ingredients that act as a stimulant in some people, so it is best to avoid using them late in the day.

Massage yourself or have a significant other do it and use an aromatherapy oil blend made up in a shop that specializes in herbs. Another alternative is a magnetic field therapy pad. This, along with massage, is relaxing, helps induce sleep, and enhances your mood and sense of well-being. This works when taking medications, when in pain, and after surgery to soothe sore bruised areas.

To prevent episodes of sleeplessness, take daytime walks outside. Light exposure during the day helps keep your body clock regulated. In fact, regular exercise late in the afternoon or in the early evening is a good way to make your body tired so that you're able to sleep more readily. If you suffer from fatigue during the day, resist the urge to take a long nap. Limit yourself to brief rest periods without prolonged sleep. Establish a regular bedtime and give yourself about 30 to 45 minutes of quiet time before you get into bed. Listen to soft music, write a letter, read, take a hot bath, or do something else that is relaxing, not stimulating. Make your bedroom a comfortable, quiet, luxurious zone by eliminating the computer, telephone, TV, fax machine, or other work-related objects. And try to confine your time for worrying to daylight hours. (Easier said than done, right?)

Remember, no matter how many hours of sleep you get each night, if you wake up easily in the morning and if you can make it through the entire day without running out of steam or feeling drowsy after sitting quietly, you are probably getting enough rest.

Medications for Anxiety, Depression, and Pain

In addition to the categories of drugs we discussed in chapter 2, there are other medications that may be part of the treatment for endometriosis to reduce anxiety, counteract depression, and help control pain. As you read the following discussion, you'll see that there are several examples in each section. Although they may generally work in the same way, there are at least minor differences between each. Why is this important? If the prescribed medication has an unpleasant side effect, there may be another drug you can take that will provide the same benefits without problems. And if the prescribed drug is not making you feel better, another medication may do the trick. Your doctor will work with you to find the medication that works best with your particular chemistry and that is compatible with other drugs you may be taking.

MEDICATIONS TO REDUCE ANXIETY

We know that endometriosis can trigger anxiety and panic. Many women can reduce these symptoms using nonpharmacological methods—relaxation techniques, exercise, and other forms of stress management. (See chapter 6 for more about anxiety.) But if medication seems to be the answer for you—especially if you've been experiencing panic attacks—there are three subcategories of drugs that may be helpful.

The first is the benzodiazepines. Examples of medications in this group include Xanax (alprazolam), Valium (diazepam), and Librium (chlordiazepoxide hydrochloride). The latter two, although able to control anxiety, are not considered as effective for panic attacks. Benzodiazepines have few side effects but can be habit-forming.

The second subcategory of drugs is the tricyclic antidepressants. These medications were actually among the earliest ones shown effective in dealing with panic, but they are now used less often, since more effective medications have been found. Examples of drugs in this category include Tofranil (imipramine hydrochloride) and Norpramin (desipramine hydrochloride).

The third subcategory is the MAO (monoamine oxidase) inhibitors, which are also antidepressants. Examples of drugs in this subcategory are Nardil (phenelzine sulfate) and Parnate (tranylcypromine sulfate). Some consider this group to be the most effective for panic control. However, of the three groups, this one probably requires the greatest attention to dosage schedules and other precautions in order to minimize side effects. For example, if you're taking a drug in this class, it is important to avoid taking antihistamines or decongestants, as the drugs might be incompatible and cause further problems. In addition, foods with high concentrations of tyramine or dopamine—aged cheeses, beer, and wine, for instance—should be avoided, as they may lead to hypertension (high blood pressure).

When using antianxiety medications, keep in mind that even when they are effective, they are really only blocking the panic attacks. It is still important to deal with the triggers of the anxiety and to implement any changes necessary to resolve the problems that led to the anxiety in the first place.

ANTIDEPRESSANTS

Unfortunately, depression is a common problem for women with endometriosis. As discussed in chapter 5, nonmedical coping techniques can help some women deal successfully with depression. When problems persist, though, antidepressants may be helpful. Examples include tricyclic antidepressants and combinations such as Elavil (amitriptyline hydrochloride), Norpramin (desipramine hydrochloride), Pamelor (nortriptyline hydrochloride), Sinequan (doxepin hydrochloride), and Tofranil (imipramine hydrochloride). Others are the MAO (monoamine oxidase) inhibitors such as Nardil (phenelzine sulfate) and Parnate (tranylcypromine sulfate). These medications work in different ways and result in different possible side effects. Other antidepressants that may be prescribed include Desyrel (trazodone hydrochloride), Prozac (fluoxetine hydrochloride), and Zoloft (sertraline hydrochloride).

PAIN MEDICATIONS

As you've discovered in chapter 12, there are several different types of techniques that can be used to control pain. Certain medications, however, are especially helpful in the relief of endometriosis-related pain.

There are a number of categories of pain control medications, also called analgesics. Two commonly used nonnarcotic pain relievers are aspirin and acetaminophen (for example, Tylenol). These medications can be very effective in relieving mild to moderate pain. Aspirin can also reduce swelling and inflammation but may affect the stomach and can interfere with blood clotting. For this reason, some women may prefer acetaminophen, even though it does not control inflammation.

Nonsteroidal antiinflammatory drugs (NSAIDs), another type of nonnarcotic analgesic, include over-the-counter, nonprescription-strength Motrin (ibuprofen), Advil (ibuprofen), Nuprin (ibuprofen), and Aleve (naproxen sodium); and prescription strength Motrin (ibuprofen), Naprosyn (naproxen), and Indocin (indomethacin). A second approved category of NSAIDs, commonly referred to as Cox-2 inhibitors, are now available for treatment of menstrual and acute pain. They have a lower risk of ulcers and bleeding from the intestinal tract than the other NSAIDs and are currently available under the brand names Celebrex and Vioxx.

Narcotic pain relievers are much more powerful than nonnarcotic analgesics. Narcotics, which are derived from opium or synthetically produced to act like drugs derived from opium, work by changing your perception of pain and creating a heightened sense of well-being. Unfortunately, these drugs can also be habit-forming and frequently cause side effects, including nausea, constipation, vomiting, or drowsiness. Examples of narcotic painkillers include codeine, Demerol (meperidine), morphine sulfate, Percodan (oxycodone/ aspirin), Percocet (oxycodone/acetaminophen), and Darvon (propoxyphene hydrochloride). These medications may be used by themselves or in combination with over-the-counter pain relievers.

Analgesics can be administered orally, in pill or liquid form; by injection; through rectal suppository; or in an intravenous drip. Pain medication can also be delivered using a pump, which can be either implanted or worn next to the body. The pain pump is commonly used to allow the self-administration of prescribed doses of powerful, fast-acting painkillers.

Whenever you deal with painkillers—as well as many other types of drugs—you have to be concerned about addiction. In fact, some people who have pain are reluctant to use painkillers because they fear addiction or because they worry that other people will think less of them for using these drugs. In general, specialists report that addiction is rarely a problem for women with endometriosis, because pain medication is usually taken only on an "as needed" basis, with the least powerful drugs being prescribed or recommended whenever possible. When the medication is no longer needed, it is discontinued.

Caution!

There is always the chance that certain drugs, including over-the-counter ones, may not be appropriate in your endometriosis treatment program. You've heard this a lot already, but it's important: check with your doctor! Question, learn, and help yourself. Consult with your physician before taking even the most innocent over-the-counter drug. You never know when you might have an adverse reaction.

In addition, be careful about bad mixes. This is so important that it bears repeating. For example, tranquilizers and alcohol should never be taken at the same time. Do not consume alcohol with acetaminophen or narcotics. Some mixes can make your symptoms worse, interfere with the action of the prescribed medication, or cause additional problems. Again, don't hesitate to ask questions!

Work with Your Pharmacist

Many people rely solely on their doctor for information about prescribed medications. If this is true of you, you're overlooking a wonderful information resource: your pharmacist. Pharmacists know a great deal about drug interactions, the foods to avoid when taking certain medications, and other possible problems or side effects. Develop a good working relationship with your local pharmacist. Compounding pharmacists can work with you to prepare medication, supplements, or hormone replacements specifically formulated for you. The International Academy of Compunding Pharmacists (IACP) offers a referral service so you can get the name of a compounding pharmacist in your area.

Besides being a good resource, your pharmacist may be able to help you reduce costs by suggesting a less expensive brand name or generic drug. While there may be nothing wrong with the substitute drug, in some cases certain formulations may work better than others. So always be sure to consult your physician before changing brands. (Depending on how your doctor filled out the prescription, your pharmacist may *have* to contact him before substituting a brand other than the one specified.) Obviously, a good relationship with a well-informed, helpful pharmacist can benefit you in more ways than one.

Additional Medication Reminders

Once you've begun taking a medication, let your physician know if the drug is having the desired effect. Report any significant changes in your health, whether good or bad. In this way, your doctor will be able to make an informed decision about whether your current drug program should be continued or changed.

If you find that you're having trouble remembering to take your medication—or if you're sometimes unsure if you've already taken a dose—find ways to keep track of your medication schedule. For instance, you might prepare a daily chart that lists each dose separately. This will allow you to check off each one as you take it. You might also purchase a multicompartment pill box, which can store a week's worth of drugs divided into appropriate days and times. Some sophisticated devices even sound an alarm when the time comes for you to pop your pill!

As previously mentioned, certain drugs are chemically incompatible with one another or may be incompatible with other aspects of your treatment. For this reason, it is essential that you put together a list of all the medications you are taking and that you keep it in your wallet. You will then be able to show the list to your doctor, your pharmacist, or anyone else who needs to know what drugs you're taking.

You may experience certain emotional reactions from some medications, such as depression or anger. Remember to learn how to cope with these responses before they adversely influence your physical and emotional well-being. If necessary, refer to the earlier chapters on coping with emotions. If the suggested strategies don't provide relief, by all means seek out a qualified professional who can help you become more comfortable with any side effects you may be experiencing as a result of your treatment plan.

A Final Prescription

Many types of drugs other than those mentioned in this chapter may also alleviate or reduce your symptoms. In fact, there are so many possible combinations of drugs that it may take your doctor a while to determine the "formula" that's best for you. Medicine is both art and science, so don't be alarmed if you and your doctor have to use a "trial and error" approach at times.

Hopefully, the information presented in this chapter has given you a good idea of what you must know in order to use medication as safely and effectively as possible. So if your doctor prescribes something new, ask about it. Not only will you probably feel a lot better as a result of taking the medication, but you'll also know *why* you're feeling better!

CHAPTER FOURTEEN

Physical Symptoms

You know better than anyone how endometriosis can affect you both physically and psychologically. We've already discussed ways to better cope with your emotions and with pain, and we've looked at ways to deal with some of the side effects from medications you may need to take. In this chapter, we'll focus on the most common physical symptoms of endometriosis and how to tackle them—problems that, as mentioned before, can play a major role in your psychological adjustment.

It is important that you know about the many different symptoms you may experience as a result of the endometriosis itself. Then they won't surprise you. Of course, you should also know about ways to control them either medically or with lifestyle changes. Might there be physical symptoms that you *can't* alleviate? Unfortunately, yes. And in that case, you'll have to learn to simply accept them. This may seem like a tall order, but what choice do you have? Try to concentrate on the things you *can* control. Deal with the symptoms as they come, if and when they come. Don't anticipate the worst, because that won't help you. It's far better to put your energy into more positive efforts.

Let's discuss some of the most common symptoms of endometriosis (other than pain) and how to deal with them. When there's something you can do, we'll give you suggestions. If no treatments or management techniques are available, you'll at least learn more about the symptoms and know that you're not alone in experiencing them.

Fatigue

Do you notice that you become tired more easily at certain times? Is bed your favorite place to be in the whole world? If so, you're not alone. Fatigue is a very common and unpleasant problem for women with endometriosis. In fact, fatigue is one of the most common symptoms of virtually every medical disorder!

You may experience fatigue while participating in some activity or after doing anything that requires energy. Or, without doing anything tiring, your body may suddenly decide it needs a rest! You may feel as if the energy has been drained right out of you, like water draining from a leaky radiator. One morning, you wake up and feel fine; then fatigue hits you unexpectedly during the day. On the other hand, you may awaken in the morning feeling very tired, and find that your energy builds as the day goes on. At certain times of the month, the fatigue may be more noticeable. For instance, many women get extremely tired two or three days before their menstrual period. Don't let it get to you. Just remind yourself that you'll be able to return to a more normal routine soon. The good news is there will be times when you are loaded with energy (for example, just after your period).

Why does fatigue occur? Fatigue may, of course, be caused by the endometriosis itself. Pain is very exhausting and can drain you of energy. Medical or surgical treatments can also sap a tremendous amount of energy, often causing both fatigue and physical weakness.

Sometimes, fatigue is totally unrelated to the endometriosis or its treatment. You may simply be doing too much! As discussed earlier in the book, psychological problems such as stress, tension, anxiety, and depression may also contribute to fatigue. Good nutrition is critical for a healthy body. Your nutritional status, poor dietary habits, and an insufficient intake of vitamins and other nutrients can make you more tired than you need to be.

Sometimes fatigue can snowball. If you're chronically tired, even a reduction of day-to-day activities may not help. Unless something happens to break the chain, you may find that you have less and less energy.

Fatigue may also result from reducing or eliminating exercise, either because you don't want to exercise or because pain makes it too difficult. But the less you do, the more out of shape and tired you'll become! (See chapter 16 for more on this topic.) So if you become fatigued on a regular basis, discuss this with your doctor. Together, you'll be able to decide what is the most likely cause and how to eliminate it.

WHAT CAN YOU DO?

Obviously the best way to cope with fatigue is to get enough rest, to ensure that your body can be nourished and heal. Allow yourself longer periods of time for sleep at night and try to arrange for at least one or two brief rest periods during the day, preferably in the late morning and late afternoon. Although this added rest may not make your fatigue disappear, it will certainly help. But remember that too much rest can actually lead to more fatigue and insomnia!

Make sure you're getting the proper amounts and types of exercise. Exercise helps to break the cycle of fatigue and poor conditioning. In fact, studies on women who experience severe fatigue as a result of radiation and/or chemotherapy demonstrate that walking is the best remedy. Though it sounds anything but restful, walking 15 to 30 minutes per day and other moderate forms of exercise decreased fatigue in these women by half. Exercise helps circulation, which in turn clears waste products from the body. It strengthens muscles and helps injured cells to heal because they get more oxygen. Another benefit of exercise is that it helps to reduce other potential causes of fatigue like depression, anxiety, and insomnia.

You can also reduce fatigue with efficient planning and pacing. Determine your exact responsibilities and schedule activities so that you won't do too many strenuous things at one time. (For more about prioritizing, refer to chapter 17.) Remember, blessed are the flexible, for they shall not be bent out of shape! Be ready to change course if fatigue hits you out of the blue, or if you have a sudden burst of energy!

In some cases, you may want to modify the activity itself. For example, perhaps you are an avid tennis player and normally spend three hours a day on the court. This may not be possible right now, so try to be satisfied with one hour instead of three.

Be willing to ask for help. Have other people accomplish some of the tasks that are lower priorities for you or that don't demand your personal attention. This will conserve your energy, allowing you to do the things that are more important.

Gastrointestinal Problems

Do you have diarrhea or severe bowel cramps around the time of your period? If so, you are not alone. Women with endometriosis often suffer from a number of gastrointestinal problems.

There are many reasons why this can happen. If there are endometrial lesions on the large intestine, you may experience painful bowel movements, a sense of rectal pressure or urgency to move the bowels, bloody stools, or even a partial obstruction (although this is a rare event). Adhesions can pull on the bowel and cause pain after exercise or intercourse or during pelvic and rectal examinations. You may also experience nausea and vomiting. But migraine headaches, medications, food allergies, and anxiety or emotional stress can also produce nausea or vomiting.

WHAT CAN YOU DO?

What can you do about gastrointestinal problems associated with endometriosis? The most important step you can take is to work with your doctor to identify the cause of your symptoms. Then he can recommend the appropriate treatment. For example, there are certain medications that relax the smooth muscles in the intestine; your doctor can prescribe one that will help reduce cramping and pain.

If you experience rectal bleeding, it is important to rule out polyps or other diseases. Your doctor may also perform a digital rectal exam or recommend that you have a diagnostic test called a colonoscopy. Be sure to contact your doctor immediately if you experience mucus or blood in the stool or frequent diarrhea.

Fortunately, there are several effective strategies to help combat diarrhea, nausea, or vomiting. Try to modify your diet. Sometimes it's the odor of food that really triggers nausea, so focus on cold foods, which usually have less odor than hot ones. Avoid places where strong-smelling food is being prepared. Dry foods, like crackers or toast, may also help. Eat smaller, more frequent meals and avoid fats, aspartame (an artificial sweetener), and monosodium glutamate (a flavor enhancer) because they can cause gastrointestinal upset, bloating, and diarrhea. Include oat bran, rice bran, yogurt, and fiber in your diet. Apples, carrots, potatoes, sugar beet, and tomatoes also help relieve diarrhea because they contain pectin, which thickens the stool.

You may be tempted to ask for your favorite foods, thinking that these will be most appealing. Be aware, though, that this isn't always the wisest strategy during bouts of nausea or vomiting. Some people find that after the nausea diminishes, they are actually turned off by former favorites!

It is important to adjust your diet to include plenty of liquids to prevent dehydration. Ginger tea is especially good. Carbonated beverages can reduce nausea, but be aware that this technique is most helpful when the beverage is allowed to stand for a while and "flatten." Avoid alcohol and medications that are known to irritate the gastrointestinal tract. You may even want to follow a liquid diet for 24 hours to give the bowel a rest.

A number of psychological techniques—including imagery, visualization, meditation, and relaxation—can reduce gastrointestinal symptoms. Acupressure and biofeedback training can also be helpful. Aromatherapy, which uses the essential oils extracted from plants and herbs, can help improve digestive function and relieve stress-related discomfort. It is ideally suited for home use. Most health food stores carry essential oils, and a practitioner is usually available to recommend specific oils that you inhale or use for massage. Chamomile, clary sage, fennel, geranium, and ginger are especially helpful for menstrual cramps and gastrointestinal pain. These essential oils are added to a carrier oil, such as sweet almond or sesame oil, and then massaged into the skin. To learn more about these techniques or products, consult a professional who is experienced with them.

If your diarrhea continues, your physician may prescribe a medication, such as Imodium (loperamide hydrochloride), Lomotil (diphenoxylate hydrochloride), or Motofen (difenoxin hydrochloride), or you can try Pepto-Bismol (bismuth subsalicylate). Antinausea and antivomiting drugs include Anzemet (dolasetron mesylate), Compazine (prochlorperazine), Kytril (granisetron hydrochloride), Phenergan (promethazine hydrochloride), Thorazine (chlorpromazine), Tigan (trimethobenzamide hydrochloride), Torecan (thiethylperazine maleate), or Zofran (ondansetron hydrochloride). Zofran, in particular, is a welcome addition to the arsenal of antinausea medications because it has fewer side effects and works well for most people. And remember that new drugs are being developed all the time.

Bladder Problems

Bladder problems are not uncommon with endometriosis, and many women are plagued by burning or pain during urination or urinary frequency. It is possible to have these types of symptoms yet not have a urinary tract infection. How can that be? Endometriosis often stretches the nerves that control blood flow to the bladder, bowel, and pelvic floor, resulting in this hypersensitivity. Or lesions can attach to the bladder or the ureter, causing all the typical symptoms of a urinary tract infection. Yeast can also cause these symptoms.

WHAT CAN YOU DO?

If you have urinary tract problems, the same steps should be followed as those already discussed: determine the cause so you can receive the appropriate treatment. If you have experienced hypersensitive bladder symptoms but haven't been diagnosed with endometriosis, a laparoscopy may be recommended. If your urine tests are "negative" for bacteria, be sure to ask your doctor to consider yeast as a possible culprit. Always consult your doctor immediately if there is blood in your urine.

Tampons, douches, bubble baths, and feminine hygiene sprays are all potentially irritating to your bladder, so don't use them. Here, again, diet modifications may help. Try drinking one-quarter teaspoon of baking soda in water or corn silk tea, which acts as a soothing coating to inflamed bladder tissue. There are many herbs and hot infusions that you can drink to help ease bladder problems. A nutritionist or herbal specialist can recommend specific combinations. Drink eight ounces of water every hour and modify your diet with foods that act as natural diuretics, such as celery, parsley, and watermelon. Avoid citrus fruits; they produce alkaline urine, which encourages bacterial growth. If you are prone to chronic bladder problems, it may be helpful to consult with a dietitian for additional diet modifications.

Heavy or Irregular Bleeding

You might find that on certain days during your menstrual period the flow is so heavy that you are scared to leave home. If you bleed through one or two tampons and a pad worn at the same time, this is considered to be heavy bleeding. Over time, it may lead to anemia (a low red blood cell count). Endometriosis can also cause you to bleed in between normal menstrual periods. However, there are other causes of heavy and irregular bleeding, such as fibroids, adenomyosis, thyroid problems, tumors, cancer, or chronic stress. Be sure your doctor rules out any of these other conditions.

WHAT CAN YOU DO?

There are several medications that will help reduce bleeding, including synthetic progestin hormones or birth control pills that regulate the menstrual cycle to control excessive bleeding. Another recommendation is natural progesterone applied to the skin or taken orally. Your dosage will depend upon the severity of the bleeding.

Prostaglandin inhibitors such as ibuprofen (e.g., Advil or Motrin), naproxen sodium (e.g., Anaprox), or mefenamic acid (Ponstel) also help decrease bleeding in some women. They are taken one or two times per day for three to four days before the menstrual cycle, through the days when the period is usually the heaviest. Endometrial ablation, cauterizing the lining of the uterus, is a surgical treatment that may be considered when other treatments fail.

Some experts suggest using physical modalities that change the electromagnetic field around the body and unblock the energy in the pelvis (such as massage, magnetic field therapy, acupuncture, and meditation). (See chapter 12 for more information.)

Once again, changes to your diet may help. Sometimes, a low-fat, high–complex carbohydrate diet reduces excessive circulating estrogen, but you should wait at least three months to see results. A dietitian can help you identify the right foods and nutritional supplements. Many general nutrition and diet books offer menu plans for low-fat, high–complex carbohydrate meals. See chapter 15 for more dietary information.

Sleep Problems

Do you toss and turn at night? Does it seem like you'll never get to sleep? Well, you're not alone! Women with endometriosis often experience sleep problems. For example, insomnia may result from pain, nausea, or other consequences of the disease. Emotions, also, may wreak havoc with your sleeping patterns. Depression, for example, often results in too much sleep, while anxiety often results in too little.

WHAT CAN YOU DO?

Obviously, if your sleep problems are rooted in emotional troubles, it is important to learn to effectively cope. And if certain symptoms related to endometriosis, such as pain or heavy bleeding, are keeping you up at night, appropriate treatment may help you get the rest you need. (For additional suggestions, see chapter 13.)

A Physical Finale

Although the physical symptoms you may experience with endometriosis are not pleasant to think about, it's important to learn as much as you can about them. You want to effectively cope with endometriosis, right? By marshaling all your forces to control these problems, you will not only improve your level of comfort but also build the confidence you need to continue leading a happy, productive life.

CHAPTER FIFTEEN

Diet

Are you eating more and enjoying it less? Research has shown that endometriosis, as well as its treatment, may affect your eating habits and, accordingly, your weight. In addition, more and more research is now focusing on a link between diet and endometriosis. Therefore, it makes sense that any woman with endometriosis should work to control her eating patterns and try to follow as healthy a diet as possible.

Why is nutrition so important, and what exactly is a good diet? Let's learn more about the role diet plays if you have endometriosis and about the changes that can help you maximize your health.

Why is Nutrition So Important?

Nutrition is the process of eating appropriate amounts of nutrients and using them to meet energy needs, to accomplish body-sustaining healing, and to satisfy maintenance requirements. Improving your nutrition is a powerful way to optimize health. The human body is very complex, but it can heal itself if you provide it with proper nourishment and care. If you do not give your body the proper nutrients, you can actually impair its normal functions and cause yourself harm. Here are just some of the benefits a sound diet may provide for the woman with endometriosis:

- A body that is well nourished is stronger than a poorly nourished one. Proper nourishment helps us fight infection, heal, and thrive.
- A good diet actually helps women respond better to endometriosis treatment and makes them more resistant to side effects.
- Eating certain foods can help alleviate many of the problematic symptoms associated with endometriosis and counteract some of the side effects of medication.
- Good nutrition provides good energy, so important because of the potential energy-zapping effects of endometriosis.
- A balanced diet increases the speed at which body tissues heal themselves.
- Without proper nutrition, the body's stores of protein, fat, vitamins, and other nutrients may be depleted. A good diet ensures continuing healthy stores of these nutrients.
- Eating healthy foods actually reduces food cravings and the urge to binge.

Dietary Recommendations

A fat-rich, fiber-poor diet may be one reason that endometriosis is on the increase, affecting millions of women. Animal fats are a major culprit because of their effects on the body's hormonal system. At this time, there is no specific "endometriosis cure diet"; however, there are some important dietary recommendations that all women with endometriosis should follow.

Perhaps it's best to begin our discussion by looking briefly at the most current dietary recommendations of the United States Department of Agriculture (USDA). If you remember the original "four basic food groups," which heavily emphasized the importance of meat, poultry, and dairy, the new guidelines may prove startling. Basing their recommendations on current research, the USDA now recommends a complex-carbohydrate, low-fat, high-fiber diet. The government has made it clear that whole grains, fruits, and vegetables are the basics of a good diet. Of lesser importance are the dairy group and the meat, poultry, and fish group. Fats, oils, and sweets, the government states, should be used only sparingly.

Certainly, the USDA guidelines make good sense for the woman with endometriosis. But let's take a closer look at some specific dietary recommendations for the woman who's learning to cope with this condition.

EAT A LOW-FAT DIET

Although this theory has not been proven, a high-fat diet may play a role in the development of endometriosis.

First, endometriosis is an estrogen-sensitive disease; excessive fat intake stimulates excess estrogen production in the body, which stimulates endometriosis—a vicious cycle! We also ingest estrogen through dietary sources (such as dairy products, beef, and eggs), giving our bodies too much of this hormone. High-fat foods, including meat, fatty fish, poultry, dairy products, and eggs can contain pollutants known as dioxins—chemical residues that may be linked to both the onset and severity of endometriosis. Dioxins are by-products of processes such as incineration, chlorine bleaching, and the use of pesticides and herbicides. Once released into the environment, they are consumed by animals. When we eat animal products, we consume dioxins, which our bodies store in fat tissues for long periods of time. It is theorized that dioxins short-circuit the body's complex hormone system and can also cause problems with the immune system, affecting antibodies and other important disease-fighting cells.

Clearly, it is wise to reduce the amount of saturated fat you eat. Following a low-fat diet has many other benefits, such as reducing the risk of developing heart disease, breast cancer, and many other disorders.

To reduce the fat in your diet, limit your consumption of red meat to about once every 10 days, and eat only lean cuts. Or you may find that eliminating red meat completely helps alleviate symptoms. Any dairy products that you consume should be nonfat or lactose-free if necessary. As much as possible, eliminate saturated oils and fats, including butter, margarine, lard, and vegetable oils. When oils can't be totally avoided, use only small amounts of polyunsaturated oils, such as peanut, canola, and safflower, or use olive oil, which is monounsaturated. Get to know the good fats—such as omega-6 fatty acids, found in nuts, wheat germ, primrose oil, borage oil, and omega-3 oils, found in salmon and mackerel. Determine which foods make you feel drained of energy or bloated or give you some other unpleasant side effect, and limit the amount of them you eat. The most common offenders are cow's milk products, food preservatives and artificial colors, wheat, chocolate, eggs, citrus fruits, and foods containing salicylates (such as apples, cherries, grapes, peaches, eggplant, broccoli, tea, and coffee).

EAT A HIGH-FIBER DIET

Some studies focus on the theory that high-fiber diets are more healthy. How does fiber protect us? Fiber—the part of plant materials that our body does not digest—binds bile acids, cholesterol, carcinogens, and other harmful substances. In other words, fiber is good for removing certain toxins from the body.

Because the refining process removes much of the natural fiber from our foods, our diet lacks this important substance. Fortunately, it's easy—and delicious—to add more fiber to your diet every day. High-fiber cereals are one of the best sources. Other good sources include brown rice, whole grain breads and pasta, bran, most fresh fruit, dried prunes, nuts, seeds, beans, unbuttered popcorn, and lentils. Raw vegetables and Brussels sprouts, broccoli, kale, and cabbage, are also rich in fiber. Eating oat bran, rice bran, apples, carrots, potatoes, sugar beet, tomatoes, and other foods high in fiber can help stop diarrhea, a common problem if you have bowel endometriosis.

EAT A DIET HIGH IN ANTIOXIDANTS

Antioxidants are a group of vitamins, minerals, and enzymes that help to protect the body from the formation of free radicals, which are atoms or groups of atoms that can cause damage to cells, impairing the immune system and leading to infections and various degenerative diseases. Antioxidants help preserve the cell's DNA, the genetic material necessary for healthy cell reproduction. Although the body makes these, there are also a number of nutrients that act as antioxidants, including vitamin A, beta-carotene, vitamins C and E, and the mineral selenium.

Women with endometriosis should regularly eat foods containing antioxidants, such as sprouted grains and fresh fruits and vegetables. Active vitamin A is found only in animal sources, such as cod liver oil, beef, and chicken. However, beta-carotene, the vitamin A precursor, is found in green and yellow-orange vegetables and fruits, including carrots, kale, kohlrabi, spinach, turnip greens, dandelion greens, apricots, and cantaloupe. Some of the foods highest in vitamin C are broccoli, Brussels sprouts, kale, turnip greens, parsley, sweet peppers, cabbage, cauliflower, and spinach. Vitamin E is found in such vegetable oils as corn, soybean, and safflower oil, and in whole grains, dark green leafy vegetables, nuts, and legumes. Selenium is found mostly in seafood and whole grains.

One final note. When adding fruits and vegetables to your diet, be sure to get the freshest produce possible, as it will have the highest levels of nutrients. Some women with endometriosis try to eat organic fruit, vegetables, and grains to reduce exposure to dioxins and to avoid the pesticides, herbicides, and other chemicals that can harm the immune system. If possible, eat the vegetables raw, as heat can destroy nutrients. When cooking vegetables, steam or microwave them briefly to preserve optimum nutrient content.

VITAMINS, MINERALS, HERBS, AND NATURAL FOOD SUPPLEMENTS

Vitamins are essential to life. They help regulate metabolism and assist the biochemical processes that release energy from digested food. Every living cell depends on minerals for proper function and structure. Minerals are needed to properly compose body fluids, form blood and bone, maintain healthy nerve function, and regulate muscle tone. Both vitamins and minerals function as coenzymes, substances that work with enzymes to enable the body to function. Many herbs and natural food supplements contain powerful ingredients that, if used correctly, can help heal the body. Because vitamins, minerals, herbs, and natural food supplements are vital to good nutrition, it stands to reason that you can benefit from a number of these if you have endometriosis.

Let's discuss vitamins and minerals first. The vitamin B complex is particularly important. This nutrient group assists estrogen metabolism and bowel function, and it helps prevent fluid retention. The B complex, as well as vitamin E and vitamin C with bioflavonoids, all help to reduce the severity of internal inflammation and to inhibit prostaglandin production. Taking a multivitamin supplement or individual doses of these vitamins can be helpful, even if you do follow a healthy diet. Minerals such as iron, calcium, magnesium, selenium, and zinc are also important. For example, iron supplements may be recommended by your doctor if you have been diagnosed with anemia. However, you should only take iron under a healthcare professional's supervision. If you are taking medication that contributes to loss of bone density, you should ask your doctor about taking a calcium, magnesium, vitamin D for- mulation. You should also ask about minerals, such as magnesium and zinc, that may help to reduce inflammation and pain, and selenium, which is known to strengthen the immune system.

What about taking herbs if you have endometriosis? Certain herbs, used in conjunction with diet, can promote health and well-being for women with endometriosis. For example, burdock root, dong quai, vitex, and red raspberry leaf help to balance hormones. Astragalus, garlic, goldenseal, myrrh gum, pau d'arco, and red clover have antibiotic and antitumor properties. Milk thistle helps support liver function and breakdown estrogen. Alfalfa is a good source of minerals, including iron. Peppermint, ginger, chamomile, valerian, and wild yam can also help certain symptoms associated with endometriosis. It is important to remember that although herbs are natural, they can be extremely toxic. Always seek the counsel of your healthcare provides or an herbal ther- apist before starting herbal therapy.

Essential fatty acids may relieve or reduce many endometriosis symp- toms, such as menstrual cramps, pain and inflammation, and hot flashes. Es- sential fatty acids such as fish oils, evening primrose, borage, and linseed oils metabolize in the body to form anti-inflammatory prostaglandins.

Remember, some physicians are not knowledgeable about vitamins, min- erals, herbs, and dietary supplements that may help with endometriosis symp- toms. Some women prefer to find a practitioner who specializes in these areas. Be sure to keep your physician informed of whatever alternative therapies you decide to use.

When choosing any type of vitamin or supplement, it is important to be aware of artificial colors, artificial flavors, synthetic sweeteners, artificial preservatives, and harsh binders and fillers. Any of these could possibly worsen your symptoms. As with any medication for endometriosis, you should review the scientific research on supplements, especially since the FDA does not regulate the industry.

AVOID HARMFUL "NONFOODS"

In addition to some of the foods you may be eating, a number of nonfoods— additives, pesticides, hormones and steroids, alcohol, caffeine, and to- bacco—can also be hazardous to your health.

Artificial Additives

Believe it or not, the average American diet includes five thousand or more artificial additives used to maintain freshness and to preserve the attractive look or taste of food. While some of these additives are safe, we don't yet know if any may be linked to endometriosis. Other additives have not yet undergone sufficient studies to determine their safety. For example, monosodium glutamate (MSG) and aspartame are used without warnings but have been known to cause a wide range of problems, including gastrointestinal upset, bloating, and diarrhea. Cyclamate and saccharine are examples of additives once deemed safe but later banned or allowed to be used only if accompanied by warnings.

What can you do to eliminate all—or at least, many—of these chemicals from your diet? Obviously, additives are most common in processed foods—canned, frozen, and prepackaged. Avoid these foods whenever you can. Instead, eat whole foods that are as close as possible to their natural state. When you do buy prepared items, choose those that have been made without additives. In addition, don't eat smoked foods (such as bacon or lunchmeats), which contain some of the most harmful processing chemicals used.

Pesticides, Steroids, Hormones

Like additives, the pesticides used to control weeds and pests are abundant in the American diet. These chemicals are found in meat, poultry, fish, dairy products, vegetables, fruits, coffee—virtually all of our foods. Many pesticides that are banned in the United States reach us through produce grown in other countries.

How can you avoid these harmful additives? Well, unless you eat only organic food that has been grown in pesticide-free soil, you consume these potentially harmful substances every day. Scrub or peel all fruits and vegetables, particularly waxed fruit. You can also clean produce with nontoxic rinsing preparations, available in health food stores. If possible, buy organically grown foods and avoid imported produce. Animals raised for human consumption are often fed steroids and hormones to induce growth. To reduce their effect, buy meats that are certified drug-free and eat less meat, eggs, and dairy products. Finally, be aware that a diet high in fiber and antioxidants can help eliminate pesticides and other harmful substances from your body.

Alcohol

Excessive alcohol consumption can exacerbate some of the problems associated with endometriosis. For example, if you are taking medications that may lead to loss of bone density, you should avoid alcohol because it can add to this loss. Alcohol is also contraindicated with many medications, especially the ones taken by many women for endometriosis pain, such as aspirin, NSAIDs, and narcotics. If you have problems sleeping, you should avoid alcohol in the evening and before bed. In addition, alcohol is known to be so damaging to the immune system that some consider it a strong immune-suppressive drug.

Is it necessary to avoid all alcohol? There's no simple answer to this question. However, it does seem wise to reduce your consumption of alcohol as much as possible. Many experts believe that one drink a day is a safe amount. Less is better. After all, you want to do all you can to make your body strong and healthy!

Caffeine

Like alcohol, caffeine—found in coffee, tea, cola, chocolate, and other foods—can increase several symptoms often experienced by women with endometriosis. It is also known to cause damage to DNA and, like alcohol, contributes to loss of bone density. Caffeine plays a strong role in PMS and will obviously exacerbate sleep problems.

Again, if you want to do everything possible to strengthen yourself, it makes sense to significantly reduce or eliminate consumption of products that contain this chemical. If you wish to drink coffee, make sure it has been naturally decaffeinated with water. And what should take the place of your coffee, tea, and caffeinated beverages? Your best bets are skim or soy milk, mineral water, unsweetened fruit juices, and vegetable juices. Besides being free of harmful caffeine, most of these drinks take a further step toward improving your health by supplying valuable nutrients.

Tobacco

Finally, we come to tobacco. By now you know that tobacco and secondhand smoke have been implicated in several life-threatening conditions, including cancer, heart disease, and stroke. Smoking also causes great damage to the immune system, and it, too, contributes to loss of bone density. Chewing to-bacco and snuff have been found to be just as harmful as cigars and ciga-rettes. Tobacco is also a stimulant and will cause sleep problems in many individuals.

In the case of tobacco, the best course of action is clear. By avoiding all tobacco—including secondhand smoke—you'll strengthen your body against not only endometriosis but also a number of other diseases.

Getting Started

Now you know why a good diet is such an important part of your treatment program. You have also learned about dietary recommendations that can help reduce the symptoms caused by endometriosis. Regardless of what stage of disease you have, you can certainly take steps that will help your body fight it. So it's time to get started—to make the changes necessary to create the healthiest diet possible! Here are a few suggestions:

- Keep a food diary and record everything you eat. This will give you a realistic look at your present diet and will suggest ways you can make improvements.

- Decrease the amount of fat you eat by limiting meat intake and in-creasing fresh fruits, vegetables, and whole grains.

- Decrease your consumption of dairy foods, and make sure that the ones you do eat are nonfat.

- Eat all foods in a form that is as close as possible to their natural state. This will maximize their vitamin, mineral, and fiber content and minimize additives.

- When possible, eat organically grown produce. When this isn't available, be sure to scrub or peel fruits and vegetables to eliminate some of the pesticides. Always peel waxed produce.

• Eat soy-rich foods. They contain phytoestrogens—natural plant compounds that act like estrogen.

• Do what you can to avoid harmful nonfoods—additives, pesticides, steroids, hormones, caffeine, alcohol, and tobacco. While you may not be able to avoid all of these substances all of the time, by cutting down on them as much as possible, you'll be doing a great deal to improve your overall health.

• Avoid "empty" calorie or "junk" foods. Cookies, potato chips, and candy, for instance, have little or no nutritional value and may keep you from eating vitamin- and fiber-rich foods. In addition, many of these foods are laden with fat.

• To help ensure an adequate intake of vitamins and minerals—especially the antioxidants—add certain ones to your dietary program. Speak to your doctor or a nutritionist about the ones that would be best for you.

• Consider taking herbs and natural nutritional supplements to help alleviate some of your symptoms or ease certain medication side effects.

• Eat regularly. If digestion is regular and frequent, your blood sugars won't fluctuate wildly and you'll enjoy greater energy and fewer mood swings. Frequent smaller meals may be the answer.

• Drink plenty of fluids, including water and organic fruit juices. Aim for 8 to 10 glasses of water each day. It will help flush out your system, assist in absorption of nutrients, maintain bowel and bladder function, and improve your overall nutritional balance and skin tone.

• Include physical activity in any dietary program. Besides toning your body, exercise before a meal can help stimulate your appetite. (See chapter 16 for more about exercise.)

- If you're suffering from nausea or loss of appetite, try eating frequent, smaller meals. (Refer to chapter 14 for more tips on fighting nausea.)

- Eat when you are hungry and stop when you are full, knowing that you can eat whenever you need to.

- Eat slowly and enjoy your food fully.

- Consider the fact that your appetite may vary depending on how you feel on any given day. During times when you're feeling better, make sure that you eat all the nutrient-packed foods you can to compensate for those times when you don't feel well.

- Stay informed! Knowing more about the link between diet and endometriosis will help you to make healthy dietary changes.

Before modifying your diet, be sure to speak to your physician or a qualified nutritionist who can offer guidance on what changes are right for you. A good nutritionist understands the biochemistry of your body and will recommend ways to balance it through the use of foods as well as vitamins, minerals, and other dietary supplements. Many of the drugs prescribed for endometriosis effect the body's supply of vitamins and minerals. Also keep in mind that, although proper diet is an important part of any treatment program—and is almost totally within your control—it is one of the most frequently ignored aspects of treatment. Nutrition is not an alternative therapy. It is fundamental to everything else you do for your body. While it is sometimes difficult to eat the right foods, isn't it encouraging to know that when you do your cells can change? Don't think that you have to completely change everything at once. Start by eating whole grains, beans, and vegetables for a month. Try to reduce meat, dairy products, caffeine, and refined foods. Or eliminate all dairy products for at least one month. Then evaluate how you feel and how your body responds. Simply decreasing the fat in your diet to 20 to 40 grams per day, without necessarily eliminating meat and dairy food, may help reduce breast tenderness, heavy menstrual bleeding, or cramps. If water retention is a problem, eat less salt and more foods that help stimulate the release of retained fluid, like asparagus, corn, grapes, cucumber, watermelon, parsley, and celery.

It may be difficult for you to change your eating habits, but once you begin to eliminate any harmful products and increase your intake of nutrient-rich foods, you're sure to feel healthier and more energetic. And you'll benefit from the peace of mind that comes from doing everything you can to help yourself. So eat healthy, eat wisely, and enjoy!

CHAPTER SIXTEEN

Exercise

In chapter 14, you learned how extra rest can help you cope with fatigue and give your body a chance to heal and "recharge." But you also learned that too much rest can make you feel more tired, leading to more rest, more fatigue, more rest. . . . Well, you get the picture! What's the solution? Exercise! The right types and amounts of exercise can help you break the fatigue–rest–fatigue cycle and make you feel better in countless other ways. In fact, working toward a higher level of fitness is one of the best ways to battle fatigue. In this chapter, you'll learn about the many benefits of exercise, and see how you—with the help of your physician or other healthcare professional—can design your own personal exercise program.

The Benefits of Exercise

Exercise is important for everyone, but especially for women who have endometriosis. By reducing fat, you may also reduce levels of estrogen and toxins, such as dioxins. This, in turn, may help reduce some endometriosis symptoms. Feeling strong and capable is essential to building health. Studies show that physically active women feel better and experience many benefits that can be helpful if you have endometriosis. Examples of these are:

- Better immune system function and lower cancer rates
- Longer life expectancy
- Less depression and anxiety
- Better mental efficiency
- More relaxation; better sleep
- Less fatigue
- More assertiveness
- Better attitude about their bodies
- Stronger bones—increased bone thickness and mass
- Stronger muscles
- Higher self-esteem

Make sure, though, that you don't do anything too strenuous without asking your doctor, nurse, or physical therapist. You want to aid progress, not inhibit it.

Exercise keeps your body trim and your muscles firm. It benefits your cardiovascular and digestive systems by helping them work more efficiently. As a result, a woman who participates in regular exercise usually has more energy, fewer physical complaints, and sleeps better than a more sedentary woman. In addition, exercise can also reduce pain and make you feel less fatigued. It has even been named as the closest thing to a "magic bullet" for maintaining youth and optimal health when used in combination with good nutrition.

Exercise is as healthy for your psychological well-being as for your body. Has your self-esteem been affected as a result of your endometriosis? Exercise can restore confidence in your body and make you feel more capable—more in control. Living with endometriosis may have also increased your level of stress. Exercise is a great release for that stress! (For many people, exercise is more calming than a tranquilizer, and it has no untoward side effects.) Through exercise, you can let off steam, relieve any boredom and frustration, and clear your mind. In fact, all of the emotions that may be troubling you—depression, anger, fear, and anxiety among them—can be controlled, either wholly or partially, through exercise. And if that's not enough of a lure, unless you exercise alone, your exercise program will lead to some healthy social interactions—which are always good for the mind!

So Why Aren't You Exercising?

Considering all the good things that exercise does, you may wonder why everybody isn't out there running, cycling, and working out. Unfortunately, many people feel that exercise is, at best, extremely boring and, at worst, very unpleasant. Only a small percentage of people really and truly enjoy regular exercise. (Are you one of them?) So the best approach is to focus on exercises—and environments—that are as pleasant as possible! This will enable you to more easily keep your commitment to your exercise program.

Then again, some women may avoid exercise not because of a lack of desire but because they find it so tiring. Or they're in so much pain that they fear that exercise will only increase their discomfort. Or perhaps they are afraid that exercise may cause additional problems. While these feelings are understandable, as we've mentioned before, as you become less and less active, your fatigue will only increase. Why? Because of deconditioning. Deconditioning—the result of inactivity—causes your muscles to grow weaker and weaker over time, giving you less and less energy. Symptoms of deconditioning include shortness of breath, rapid heartbeat, and increased fatigue. Fortunately, deconditioning can gradually be reduced through regular exercise. By embarking on a gradually building exercise program, you can slowly increase your ability to participate in these activities. How can you begin? Stay tuned!

Getting Started

Before beginning any exercise program you should, of course, consult with your physician. He will probably either prescribe a treatment program herself or refer you to a physical therapist or exercise trainer.

Next, commit yourself to a regular routine. There is no benefit to exercising for a day or two and then giving up. If you want to feel better, you'll have to exercise regularly. Make it a priority three times a week! But be patient. Most exercise programs really don't show results for three or four weeks or more. But as long as you stick to it, you will see results.

Anybody who attempts to accelerate an exercise program to bring about faster results will end up suffering—and, possibly, abandoning it. So implement your routine gradually. In fact, the longer it's been since you've done any exercise, the slower your return should be.

Expect the first few weeks to be the most difficult, since your muscles may be out of shape and need time to regain their strength. So expect increased fatigue for a while, as well as a few new aches and pains. These temporary discomforts are perfectly normal and will disappear as you consistently participate and gradually increase your exercise. How often must you exercise in order to reap the many benefits? Usually, three or four times a week, for a minimum of 20 minutes each time, is needed to recondition your body. However, some people have found that they feel best when they exercise five or six times a week. Gradually, you'll find out what works for you.

Exercising Caution

We've already mentioned the importance of working with a physician, physical therapist, or other healthcare professional when starting an exercise program. This will not only ensure that the program you've chosen is safe but will also give you a "partner" in your program—someone who will help you keep track of what you're doing and of how it's helping you. If you're working with a health spa or club, you should, of course, inform the staff of your condition. But remember that they are not healthcare professionals or experts in endometriosis! So be sure to check on any exercise program recommended by the club with your doctor. If you have had surgery recently, you may be restricted for a short period of time. Find out what you can do as an alternative so that you regain your strength and don't take two steps back. Even after major abdominal surgery, walking is the first activity that physicians recommend.

It's also vital to exercise properly, following appropriate guidelines and safety rules. Again, do not force yourself. You'll want to follow a concept known as the "progression principle," which states exercise should be started slowly and, as time goes by, increased in intensity.

We mentioned earlier that you should expect to feel more aches and pains as you begin your program. But it's important to learn the difference between muscle soreness, which is probably a normal response to exercise, and acute pain. Acute pain may mean that you're overdoing it or that you're participating in an exercise that's not appropriate. The old saying "No pain, no gain" is not true when you have endometriosis. So if the discomfort you feel is extreme, by all means stop exercising and consult with a professional. You may have to choose a different form of exercise or otherwise modify your routine.

One last caution is in order. Sometimes the pain of endometriosis can be so uncomfortable that you just may not be able to exercise. Don't feel guilty about this, and don't try to force yourself if you're really not up to it. Rest as long as necessary, and be assured that you will eventually be able to resume your exercise routine.

Categories of Exercises

While all exercises work to improve stamina and muscle tone, there are other benefits as well. Different exercises achieve different goals. Most exercises belong in one of four groups: stretching; aerobic or endurance; muscle strengthening; and range of motion. Which types should you choose? Well, it's usually important to include exercises that will maintain muscle tone, normal joint motion, and overall fitness. Of course, your choice will depend partly on your own specific goals and on your own preferences.

Remember, though, that how regularly you perform your exercise routine is more important than the type of exercise. Consistency and persistence are the keys to improving your strength, endurance, flexibility, and general well-being. And combining regular exercise with proper nutrition makes good sense.

When beginning your exercise program, be careful not to overdo. Depending on your treatment and your current level of fitness, consider starting with a sustained five- or ten-minute effort. Gradually increase this time as you feel stronger and have more confidence.

Aerobics, such as brisk walking, step exercises, jogging, riding a regular or stationary bicycle, climbing stairs, using a treadmill, dancing, and swimming are all wonderful examples of ways to keep fit. Heel-to-toe walking is a style of walking that involves your whole body in one gliding, heart-pumping, joint-flexing, muscle-working, calorie-burning motion. It is ideally suited for women with endometriosis because it not only tones muscles but stretches your joints and provides the weight-bearing exercise that helps protect bone density. An even better benefit is the therapy it provides the spirit—it can give you a sense of mastery and self-esteem as you learn and perfect your technique.

KEGEL EXERCISES

Kegel exercises help strengthen pelvic floor muscles, enhancing sexual performance and pleasure. Because women with endometriosis often have urinary frequency and other bladder problems, it is important to improve the muscle tone of the bladder. To do these exercises, first you must locate your pelvic muscles. There are several ways to feel where they are and what it feels like to tighten them:

- When you are urinating, try to stop and start the stream.
- Tighten your rectal muscles as if you are trying not to pass gas. Then, if you can, try to shift the tightness from the rear to the front of your bottom area.
- Tighten your vaginal muscles around an object such as one or two inserted fingers, a tampon inserted halfway, a dildo, or a man's penis during intercourse.

To do the exercises, begin by emptying your bladder. Then try to relax completely. Tighten the muscles and hold for a count of 10, then relax the muscle completely for a count of 10. You should feel a sensation of lifting of the area around your vagina or of pulling around your rectum. Do 10 exercises in the morning, 10 in the afternoon, and 15 at night. Or you can exercise for 10 minutes three times a day. These exercises can be practiced anywhere and anytime. Most women find that these exercises are relaxing and easy to perform.

General Exercise Guidelines

It is good to keep in mind a few general guidelines that will help you derive the greatest benefits from your exercise program—without straining your muscles or worsening your symptoms. Some of the following points have not yet been mentioned in this chapter. Others have already been discussed, but they are important enough to bear repeating.

- Don't wait until your endometriosis symptoms disappear before starting an exercise program! Get involved in exercises that will help you feel better now.
- Check with your physician or other healthcare professional before starting any exercise program.
- Begin every exercise routine with a short warmup, using stretching exercises to limber the muscles, preparing the body for the more strenuous activities to follow.
- Develop your ability to tolerate exercise slowly. Too rapid an increase or too intense a program may only worsen the pain—as well as lessen your desire to exercise.
- Anticipate minor discomforts during your first days or weeks. If the pain or discomfort seems excessive or lasts too long, tell your doctor or other professional. You're probably overdoing it. Always listen to your body!
- Rather than exercising whenever the spirit moves you, set aside a regular time each day or several days a week for your exercise routine. Then stick to your schedule and make it a priority!
- Don't compare your exercise program with somebody else's. Remember that your own situation—your special needs and limits—is unique.
- Select the exercises that you enjoy or at least can tolerate.
- Commit to an exercise program for at least two months.
- Remember that exercise instructors may know very little, if anything, about endometriosis. So first check all of their suggestions with your doctor.
- Combine exercise with good nutrition.
- For muscle cramps, tightness, or discomfort after exercise, treat yourself to a hot bath, a massage, or a sauna and drink plenty of water.

A Final Exercise

Exercise can be extremely valuable or extremely harmful—or anything in between—depending on the care you use in choosing and following your program. Because every woman with endometriosis is different, there is no one set of exercises that can be recommended for everyone. But everybody is capable of doing some exercises, and can benefit from them. Just don't jump in feet first! Use your head. Speak to your physician—or, perhaps, to a physical therapist who's in touch with your physician. Then start slowly, build up your stamina, and enjoy your improved health!

CHAPTER SEVENTEEN

Activities

What can you do, what can't you do? Sure you have endometriosis, but what does this mean in terms of the basic activities in your life? Even if you feel fine, you may be nervous about participating in any vigorous activities. You may want to minimize the strain you put on your body. Then again, you may be in so much pain that you can't even consider engaging in your usual activities!

Every woman is different. You may feel exhausted most of the time, especially if you have chronic fatigue syndrome. Your current physical condition is also an important factor. For example, if you're in pain, you may want your doctor to give you the green light (or even a cautious yellow) to continue "doing your thing."

Let's discuss various activities and what, if any, effects endometriosis may have on your ability to participate in them.

Working

Working is very important for many women. It helps promote independence and provides a sense of self-fulfillment and self-worth. Of course, working also provides financial security because of the income it generates. And it is an important component of your social life. Understandably, you are probably quite concerned that endometriosis may interfere with work. Let's look at some specific job-related concerns.

SHOULD YOU CONTINUE WORKING?

While some women with endometriosis are eager to remain on the job, others question whether or not they *should* work. What's the answer? If you want to, you need to, and you can, then you should! Of course, you may have to make some modifications to avoid severe fatigue. And there may be times when you need some time off because of pain, other symptoms, or treatments. As you might suspect, it would be best to consult with your doctor regarding any job-specific limitations or restrictions you should heed.

WHAT IF PAIN OR OTHER DISCOMFORTS ARE A PROBLEM?

You may be concerned that symptoms or treatment side effects will prevent you from adequately performing your job. Certainly, endometriosis may affect your productivity—especially if your treatment is not controlling your symptoms as well as you'd like it to. You may feel that you just don't have the stamina necessary to perform satisfactorily. Your work rate may have slowed down, and you may be absent or late more than usual. If your employer is aware of any of these problems, you may have fear—that your job is in jeopardy.

What should you do? Pace yourself. Take rest breaks whenever necessary—and possible—to improve your comfort and productivity. If you've recently had surgery, don't expect too much all at once. Do what you can, and let your body be your guide.

What's the best approach if you have to shorten your hours or modify your work in some way? Well, be aware that employers are not required by law to make any special provisions for you because you have endometriosis. You still have to do what your job description details. If you're a valued employee, your company may be willing to make any minor modifications necessary to retain your services.

Of course, you might feel uncomfortable about approaching your employer. It may bother you to seek "special treatment." But consider that any necessary modifications may be small in comparison to the ones your company would face if they had to hire a new employee to replace you!

Dora had been working in the same office for 18 years. Lately, though, because of endometriosis, she had been having more difficulty completing her responsibilities and getting to work on time. Unfortunately, her supervisor was a perfectionist who apparently was unwilling to accommodate Dora's needs. She gave her a review and made it perfectly clear that unless her performance and attendance improved, she would be dismissed. As if that wasn't bad enough, the supervisor frequently reminded Dora that she was watching her. The pressure became so hard to bear that it began to affect Dora's emotional and physical health.

What if your employer is not flexible? What if you are given an ultimatum that if productivity does not improve, you will be discharged? If this happens, simply do the best you can. Consider having your physician contact your supervisor or preparing a letter that explains your limitations. If your employer doesn't understand enough about endometriosis to know that you must pace yourself and shows little or no willingness to cooperate, then you're probably better off not working there.

You should be aware that, in some cases, even if your employer is willing to accommodate you, union rules and state labor regulations can prohibit exceptions. In some states, hourly employees must make up lost hours within a certain time frame or those hours are considered overtime. There may also be restrictions on "comp" time for salaried employees.

What if another employee resents any special treatment you've been given? Try to sit down, one-on-one, and have a conversation with your unhappy colleague. Explain your situation as much as necessary. Often this is all that's needed to bring about greater understanding and cooperation. If your coworker still doesn't understand, content yourself with knowing that you tried. Now it's her problem! (For more information on dealing with colleagues, see chapter 19.)

SHOULD YOU DISCUSS YOUR CONDITION WITH YOUR EMPLOYER?

Obviously, some employers will be very supportive and understanding of your condition, while others may be somewhat apprehensive about retaining—or hiring—you because you have endometriosis. Try to reassure your employer that you'll make every effort to keep your condition from interfering with your ability to get the job done. The reality is that most women with endometriosis can fulfill work obligations much the way anybody else can! If, at some point, modifications do have to be made, you'll deal with them—and your employer—at that time.

WHAT IF EMPLOYERS REFUSE TO RETAIN OR HIRE YOU?

Employers may be hesitant to retain or hire a woman with endometriosis for a number of reasons. For instance, an employer may feel that health insurance premiums will be much higher if you are listed on the plan or even that the insurance carrier will cancel the existing coverage. But don't accept this argument. The Americans with Disabilities Act (ADA), most recently amended in 1994, clearly states that any employer with 15 or more employees must not refuse you appropriate work or discriminate against you because of any disability. Endometriosis, as well as other diseases, may be considered a disability.

While the ADA was originally passed with the intent of providing access and employment opportunities to the physically and mentally disabled, it has since been extended to cover a number of ailments. The ADA defines "disability" as any one of the following three categories: a physical or mental impairment that substantially limits one or more of the major life activities of the individual; a record of such impairment; or being regarded as having such an impairment. Most women with endometriosis would easily qualify under the first definition. The second definition is also important because it emphasizes the need to document, preferably by regular physician visits and treatment history, the progression of your disease and its symptoms. The ADA addresses both the hiring process and the employer's obligations to an employee with a disability. The law mandates that an employer must not discriminate against a person with a known disability who is "otherwise qualified" for a job and capable of performing its "essential functions" with or without "reasonable accommodations." Employers must not make employment decisions (hiring and firing) on the basis of a person's disability and must provide "reasonable accommodations" to those employees with disabilities.

What does all this mean in reality? If during the course of an interview, a prospective employer asks you about your health and you reveal your history with endometriosis, including the fact that in the past or in the future you may require some special accommodations, failure to hire you may be discrimination if the health issue was the reason for not hiring you. On the other hand, if you are already employed, firing you because of your medical condition may be illegal. However, the law does allow employers to reassign an employee to a lower-paying position after a leave of absence for treatment of a disability. And the courts generally side with employers on the issue of poor attendance as a reasonable accommodation. But the employer's attendance policy must be applied equally to all employees.

If you are denied a job or dismissed from your present one because of endometriosis, don't take it sitting down. Instead, call someone! For example, contact state authorities or the Equal Employment Opportunity Commission (EEOC)—dial 1-800-669-4000, and you'll be directed to the branch nearest you. Or check into resources such as your local bar association, which can direct you to an attorney who can help enforce the terms of this legislation. Be sure to ask for a list of attorneys who specialize in employment law and/or offer free or discount consultations. Don't let a lack of financial resources keep you from making sure that your rights are protected!

WHAT ABOUT RETURNING TO WORK?

If you have had surgery for endometriosis, your return to work will be a very important step, not only for you but for your family members as well. All of you will feel that life is returning to a more normal state.

Some women are ready to return to work as soon as they feel better. What you choose to do should depend on you, your doctor, your employer, and the nature of your work. If you are apprehensive about your return, have confidence in yourself. The more positive your attitude is and the better you present yourself, the more quickly you'll adjust.

WHAT IF YOU HAVE TO CHANGE JOBS?

If you're experiencing limitations, your old position may no longer be right for you. If this is the case, you should certainly consider transferring to another job, even if it means getting additional training.

Lori had been working as a nurse's aide, but her doctors felt she shouldn't continue doing this type of work because it was too strenuous. Lori became very depressed and unsure of what other possible job she might pursue and enjoy. She was afraid that any new training might be too difficult. Rather than face the prospect of being unable to work, Lori shut down emotionally. Fortunately, a good friend gave her some ideas that allowed her to use her skills in another way. She was given the job of training nurse's aides in the same facility where she had previously worked. Lori was happy to still be among the coworkers she liked so much and was able to bring her old skills to her new job.

Certainly the prospect of having to look for work is more daunting to some than to others. But if for any reason you are unable to continue in your present job, don't despair. There are many ways you can get the training you need to move into a different position. Your first step might be to check with any of the government services that offer vocational counseling. Counselors in these offices will work with you to determine your aptitude for different jobs. You will then be able to get the training and support you need to find employment in another field. Your state employment services may be a good place to start, especially since these services are available free of charge. In addition, the Federal Rehabilitation Act of 1973 requires states to include individuals in vocational rehabilitation programs if their previous jobs are no longer appropriate for them. These programs vary, so it's important to check with your state's Office of Vocational Rehabilitation to find out what's available. Any financial advisor you're working with should also be able to help you in this regard.

You may feel that, for financial reasons, you should postpone looking for a new job until your old one has been terminated. This tactic has its pros and cons. If you receive unemployment benefits for losing your job, this could ease your financial burden. But if subsequent employers are reluctant to hire you because of the grounds for your dismissal, this tactic may backfire. You are the only one who can decide which course of action is best for your unique needs.

IS WORKING YOUR ONLY OPTION?

As you know, there are many benefits to working, including satisfaction, pride, and money. But a paying job is not the only type of gratifying work that's available. Many meaningful, productive activities can be pursued on a voluntary basis. Check with nonprofit charities, religious and political groups, hospitals, schools, senior citizen centers, and the like. These organizations, and many more, can always use some extra help. For example, working with groups like the Endometriosis Research Center or the Endometriosis Association makes many women feel that they are fighting endometriosis through helping others with the disease. Volunteer work may even allow you to explore new areas of interest you couldn't pursue because of work commitments. And this will help you feel good about yourself in the bargain.

What if you just don't want to work? If this is your preference, and you're able to manage without a job, that's great. But don't use your condition as an excuse for not working. Instead, try to find out what's really bothering you and explore ways to cope with these issues.

School

Teenagers and young women with endometriosis may have problems in school that are similar to those experienced by women who work. There may be times when your condition just doesn't allow you to feel comfortable enough to attend classes. Or you may be concerned because pain prevents you from participating in your usual activities. When necessary, you should inform your teachers about your condition so that they can help whenever possible. For example, if you know that you will be having severe menstrual pain and may miss an examination or a deadline for an assignment, don't wait until after the fact to discuss it. Be honest and explain your concerns in advance so that you may be granted an extension or be allowed to take a makeup exam. (More information on children or adolescents with endometriosis can be found in chapter 25.)

Recreation

As we've mentioned in earlier chapters, you should continue to pursue the activities you've always enjoyed. Physical activities may help keep you limber and vigorous and even offer pain relief. Just as important, they will provide a welcome diversion from any worries, prevent boredom and depression, and, very likely, bring you in contact with other people.

Fortunately, most women with endometriosis are able to participate in their normal recreational activities. What you do or don't do will depend solely on your own condition and, of course, on the recommendations of your doctor. If your doctor has given you the green light, and you try an activity without experiencing excessive pain, fatigue, or other problems, you can feel confident that this activity is okay. On some days, of course, this same sport or pastime may prove to be too much for you. Again, as long as your doctor has given approval, let your body be your guide.

The Activities of Daily Living

Among the things you do each day are numerous routine tasks, what we call the activities of daily living. Of course, any symptoms you're experiencing because of endometriosis may now be limiting these activities. For many women, the symptoms of endometriosis appear long before they are officially diagnosed. If this is true in your case, you're probably experiencing a lot of frustration, and you may be just too uncomfortable, depressed, or upset to look for a creative solution to these day-to-day challenges.

Below are some practical suggestions to help you reorganize your lifestyle, household, work environment, and activities in a way that will lessen your difficulties and salvage a lot of your dignity.

SIMPLIFY YOUR TASKS

When learning to cope with routine activities, keep in mind that your goal is to make daily living as easy as possible in order to conserve energy and increase your comfort. Reduce or eliminate those activities that aren't necessary, and simplify those that are. This will leave you with more energy for the things you need—or want—to do.

In many cases, various healthcare professionals will be able to help you solve any problems you may experience when performing ordinary tasks. But it can also be very satisfying to develop your own solutions to these problems. Begin by evaluating everything you do on a day-to-day basis. Then see how you can make every single thing you do easier. Is this taking the lazy way out? Of course not. You're simply recognizing that every bit of energy you save in the performance of one activity will give you more energy with which to do something else.

Try reorganizing your home and habits so that movement becomes easier and frequently used items are within easy reach. There are a number of different gadgets that may make life more comfortable for you, including devices that will enable you to reach items high up on shelves or down near the floor without stretching or bending.

PLAN AND ORGANIZE YOUR ACTIVITIES

In addition to eliminating unnecessary activities and making the remaining tasks easier to accomplish, you'll want to learn how to use planning and pacing to conserve energy. Try charting your activities, including both your required tasks and your optional social and leisure activities. This may help you better organize your time. The further in advance you plan, the better—especially when big projects are involved—as this will give you time to figure out exactly how you're going to perform a given task, what equipment you'll need, and how to pace yourself, if necessary, to allow for rest periods. Your local library and bookstores should have some excellent books on time management. Many of the tips in these books make such good sense that you'll probably wonder why you didn't think of them yourself! And every bit of time you save will be a big plus.

A Final Exertion

By now you've learned a lot about coping with endometriosis, and you know that staying active is just as important as any other strategy. We all want to feel productive and enjoy life. Don't let endometriosis confine you to your bed or chair. Certainly you should modify any activities that are causing you discomfort, but the important thing is to do as much as you can!

CHAPTER EIGHTEEN

Financial Problems

Coping with the medical costs of any chronic illness can eventually take a financial toll. Bills for doctor's visits, laboratory tests, hospitalizations, surgery, medications, and other medical services all add up. Lost earnings may add to the financial burden if you find you can work only part-time or you must give up work altogether. Certainly, the cost for each woman—as well as the sources of these costs—varies considerably. But it may not take long for financial security to turn into financial troubles.

Let's take a look at the many ways you can prevent or ease financial problems as you cope with endometriosis.

Talk to Others

If mounting medical expenses threaten to engulf you, perhaps the first thing you should do is speak to other women with endometriosis. Through a support group, for instance, you may meet others in similar situations. Find out what they have done to control and meet the costs of their own care. Even though you may initially be embarrassed to bring up this subject, the common bond that exists among people with medically induced financial problems should quickly put you at ease. You'll be glad you brought it up!

For more ideas, you might contact your physician, hospital administrators, and other health professionals, social workers, and various organizations, such as the Endometriosis Research Center or the Endometriosis Association. Through these contacts, you will be able to find out about certain benefits and how to apply for them. You may be eligible for disability payments (if you have a policy that covers this). Even though you are not poverty-stricken, your medical bills alone may qualify you for medical assistance (Medicaid). You will need to determine the requirements for the state where you live because Medicaid coverage varies.

Your physician might also be able to prescribe less expensive treatment. For example, you could use a GnRH agonist in nasal spray form rather than receiving a monthly injection, which adds the cost of the office visit to that of the drug. And there are a few very conscientious surgeons who will reduce their fees for a woman in great need. So always talk to your physician openly and honestly if you have financial concerns.

Lower Medication Costs

If your treatment includes medication, the use of generic drugs may save you money. Generic medication is sold by its chemical name rather than the more common brand name and is usually less expensive. Ask your physician if you can take the generic versions of any drugs you're currently using. If so, your doctor will let your pharmacist know that he has okayed the substitution. Be sure to check with your pharmacist; not all generics may have the same therapeutic response as their brand-name counterparts.

Some pharmaceutical manufacturers have programs to help make some drugs available free of charge to needy patients. These are known as "indigent patient drug programs" and are available through your physician. To qualify you must have low income and no health insurance. Your doctor or nurse will contact the pharmaceutical company and request an application, which you must complete and then have your doctor authorize.

Attend a Clinic

If medical costs are overwhelming you, consider attending a clinic for medical care. Because clinics usually operate on a sliding fee schedule, you may be able to receive quality medical care at a reduced cost. In some cases, you may even be able to continue seeing the physician who's treating you now, since many physicians see patients in hospital clinics as well as in their offices. A physician may not accept your insurance in his office, but you could be treated by the same doctor in an alternative setting, such as a hospital outpatient center.

Linda, a 41-year-old consultant, wanted a second opinion and learned the name of a specialist who was highly recommended. Unfortunately, she found out that her insurance was not accepted in his office. However, her insurance *was* accepted in the outpatient clinic of a major teaching hospital where he saw patients on scheduled days. So Linda saw him in that setting rather than his private office. Although medical students, interns, and residents were involved in her care, the doctor she wanted was the "main man," and Linda made sure that he was the one who performed her surgery. The bottom line? Linda received full coverage under her insurance plan, with no additional out-of-pocket costs, and also benefited from the best surgeon in her area.

Ask your local hospital or your physician to guide you to a good clinic in your geographic location that has the resources you need.

Insurance Can Be an Assurance

Fortunately, many women have some or most of their medical costs defrayed by insurance. Even if you have health insurance, though, endometriosis can be a costly disease. That's all the more reason to get the best insurance coverage possible. For instance, tell your employer how important it is to have a healthcare plan that allows you a choice of physicians. There are too few endometriosis specialists; a plan that provides many benefits but does not allow you to see a specialist will not be very helpful for you. Insurance policies do cover a number of medical costs. However, you may have difficulty getting reimbursement for certain aspects of living with endometriosis. For example, some medical plans require that all noninvasive treatments be tried before they will approve invasive "elective" surgery. This is particularly true for hysterectomy and surgeries involving female reproductive organs.

Most insurance policies have a deductible—an amount of money you must pay before the insurance coverage begins. In addition, you may have to pay a small percentage of all costs (known as a coinsurance or copayment), with the insurance company picking up the rest of the tab.

GETTING THE MOST FROM YOUR INSURANCE POLICY

If you have a health insurance policy, contact your agent or company benefits manager as soon as possible and find out as much as you can about the benefits. (The policy itself will provide this information, too, of course.) It is important to know the amount of your deductible; the number of covered hospital days and the amount paid per day; the coverage provisions for surgery and anesthesia; payment for second opinions; and the maximum lifetime coverage allowed. Also make sure you know all of the procedures necessary to obtain a referral, file a claim, and submit an appeal.

How can you help ensure that the process of claim filing and reimbursement runs smoothly? If you are responsible for the payment of your insurance premiums, make sure you pay them on time. Don't allow your policy to lapse. Also be sure to keep track of paperwork. Every time you send in a claim, keep copies of the claim form and of any doctors' bills for your own files. These may prove invaluable if a problem arises in the processing of your claim. If, in fact, you do not receive reimbursement within 60 days, follow up by phone or letter and request an explanation if the company has denied payment. If you don't receive a satisfactory response, contact the insurance commissioner of your state, requesting an investigation.

Also keep records of the amount your insurance company pays on each claim, as well as what you pay. Your out-of-pocket payments may be deductible on your next income tax return. (Your accountant should be able to provide more information on this.)

WHAT IF YOU LEAVE YOUR JOB?

In the past, when people left jobs (either voluntarily or nonvoluntarily) they also lost the health insurance that was included with that job. Fortunately, a federal law called the Consolidated Omnibus Budget Reconciliation Act (COBRA) has changed this. Under the law, your employer has to allow you to keep your existing health insurance policy with the same coverage for up to 18 months after you leave. You will have to pay for this coverage, and it may cost you more than when you were working, but it's better than not having any insurance.

WHAT IF YOUR INSURANCE IS INADEQUATE?

If your health coverage is exhausted or your insurance is simply not good enough, you may be able to increase the ceiling for your coverage. Additional insurance may also be available for "catastrophic" medical expenses. Be aware, though, that women with endometriosis may have difficulty obtaining additional health or disability insurance. For example, a disability plan may exclude you from coverage for a period of two or more years if you have surgery or any expenses related to this condition. However, a good insurance agent can work with you to get this exclusion time reduced with supporting medical documentation. Be persistent! It's important to fight any insurance discrimination. This can take the form of canceled coverage, reduced benefits, increased premiums, or loss of insurance because of employment termination.

WHAT IF YOU HAVE NO HEALTH INSURANCE?

If you are not presently covered by health insurance, you'll want to immediately contact all your resources—your accountant, your lawyer, your financial advisor, and organizations such as the Endometriosis Research Center or the Endometriosis Association, for instance—to learn about available options. The more individuals you contact, the more likely it is that you'll find the information you need. Of course, if you are unable to obtain coverage and can't afford to pay your medical costs, you may be able to obtain assistance from government programs.

Government Programs May Help

Government insurance programs are an important source of financial support for many people. Let's take a look at three programs that may prove helpful to you.

MEDICARE

Medicare, a federal health insurance program, provides coverage for Americans age 65 and over and for disabled people of any age who qualify for and receive social security disability insurance (SSI). The degree of coverage provided by Medicare varies widely, so it's vital for you to determine exactly what health services Medicare will cover in your case. There are two forms of Medicare—traditional and Medicare+Choice.

Traditional Medicare is divided into two parts. Part A covers hospitalization and inpatient services in a skilled nursing facility, home health services, and hospice care. No premiums are required for part A insurance. Part B covers doctor's charges, outpatient hospital services, and specified medical items and services not covered under part A. Unlike part A, part B is voluntary and requires you to enroll and pay a monthly premium. In addition, part B requires an annual deductible and a 20 percent copayment on your part.

Medicare+Choice offers other ways to receive traditional medical benefits and other services through managed care plans, medical savings accounts, and preferred provider organizations.

Enrollment in Medicare is automatic upon your application for monthly social security benefits at age 65. If you decide to continue working past the age of 65, you must apply separately for Medicare. Remember, though, that while Medicare does provide coverage for large costs, it will not cover everything. Especially in the case of a major illness, supplementary medical coverage is vital.

MEDICAID

Medicaid can offer benefits to individuals who are unable to pay for health care. This public assistance program is administered on the state or local level. Who qualifies for Medicaid? Individuals who demonstrate need (e.g. very low income, high medical expenses) may be eligible. If you have any questions about qualifications or about the benefits themselves, check with your state office of health services for further information.

SOCIAL SECURITY DISABILITY INSURANCE

Disability benefits are included in the Social Security Act. A person is considered to be "disabled" if she is unable to do any substantial gainful work because of a physical or mental impairment; and if the physical or mental condition is expected to last, or has lasted, for at least 12 months or is expected to result in death. Your eligibility for this coverage will also depend on the stage and site of your endometriosis. If you are eligible for these benefits, you will receive a fixed monthly benefit, calculated the same way—and equaling the same amount—as your retirement benefits. Your local social security office should be able to tell you if you're eligible for disability insurance. The Endometriosis Association can also provide important tips if you are thinking of applying for disability.

A Final $ummation

Financial concerns can be a big worry, but despite high costs, most women are able to find ways to pay for appropriate treatment. The earlier you start planning, and the more qualified professionals you consult, the greater the likelihood that medical costs will not become a major burden. You will then be able to concentrate on your most important goal: living successfully with endometriosis.

Interacting with Other People

CHAPTER NINETEEN

Coping with Others—
an Introduction

You do not live your life in isolation—unless you're reading this book on a deserted island in the South Pacific! Because you interact with many people every day, you'll certainly want to learn how to deal with any difficulties in your interpersonal relationships. For example, you might be worried about what others are going to think when you talk about endometriosis, the pain you are experiencing, or any other symptoms. How are they going to react? Are they going to ask questions or assume that you are exaggerating? Which answers will help them to understand what you are experiencing, and which ones will turn them away?

Obviously, different problems exist in different relationships. Before we begin discussing all the various people who may be part of your life, here are a few general guidelines you may find helpful.

Do Unto Others . . .

When you interact with others, try not to be too focused on your own feelings. Disregarding the feelings of others will prevent them from getting close to you. So make a conscious effort to be considerate of others, just as you'd like them to be considerate of you.

What does this mean? Just this: *You're not the only one who has to cope with endometriosis.* The important people in your life may also be having a hard time, simply because you mean a lot to them. Remember that. You might not realize that your problems affect those around you. You might think, "Why would they be upset? It's happening to me!" But if you give this some thought, you'll see that you're not being reasonable or fair.

Take your family, for example. A problem for you is also a problem for them. Of course, it may affect you in a different way. It's certainly true that you're the one who's experiencing the pain, as well as the apprehensions and anxieties, but your family doesn't like to see you suffer. You'll be better able to cope with these important people if you bear in mind that they are experiencing almost as much emotional turmoil as you are. In fact, this may explain why family members and friends might be unable to provide all of the support you want as quickly as you would like it. This is a tough period of adjustment for everyone involved.

Perhaps you feel guilty about the added burden you are placing on your family. It can be difficult to cope with this feeling. Keep in mind, though, that you may be projecting this attitude onto your loved ones—and possibly adding to their problems in the process. Chances are, they don't feel as burdened as you may fear. They may feel temporarily helpless or overwhelmed but still be eager to help.

Change Yourself, Not Others

Do you feel that if you try hard enough, you'll be able to change the attitudes, feelings, or behaviors of others? Unfortunately, it doesn't work that way. Whether the people in your life accept your endometriosis or deny that you have any problem at all, you may have a problem changing their thinking. Instead, use your energy to change the one person over whom you do have control—yourself. Spend more time working on yourself and less time worrying about others. In fact, once others see the changes in you, they may even alter their own attitudes.

Learn to Say "No"

Perhaps you've been feeling rotten, but others are demanding your time and attention. In the past, you may have had trouble saying "no"—because you felt guilty, perhaps, or because you wanted to avoid disappointing the other person. But now things are a little different, and you really must curtail your generosity for the sake of your own well-being. Yes, this may give you the appearance of being selfish. But as long as you don't abuse it, this selfishness can be positive for you. Do for yourself; think of yourself. You're Number One, and that's the way it must be. Only if you take care of yourself will you be able to deal with others. The reverse does not necessarily hold true. If you always take care of others first, this may actually make you less able to care for yourself.

Develop a Strong Support System

You'll find it far easier to deal with endometriosis if you can rely on those closest to you, such as your spouse, other family members, and close friends. A strong social network can give you added strength in dealing with this disease.

However, it's up to you to decide how to discuss your endometriosis with others. With many medical conditions no one ever needs to be the wiser; on the other hand, is there really something wrong with people knowing you have this disease? There's nothing to be ashamed of. Endometriosis is part of you, just as the color of your hair or eyes is part of you. In addition, there may be a time that you experience an endometriosis-related problem or emergency and you need somebody who understands this disease and can help you.

Another advantage to telling friends about endometriosis is that you won't feel different when you are with them. If they know about your disease and they accept you, it will be less of an interference. They'll view you simply as a member of their circle of friends, relatives, or acquaintances, just as they always have. In addition, their knowledge of your condition will allow them to provide needed encouragement when you're feeling down.

If you decide that you want to start being more open about your illness, determine whom you want to talk to, what you're going to say, and how you're going to say it. You don't have to go into extended detail. You don't have to provide more information than they need or want. Showing how well you're coping will help them adjust.

Open the Lines of Communication

We've just discussed how the support and understanding of others can help you deal with your endometriosis-related problems. But right now, you may find it difficult to even talk to others. So how can you possibly ask for their support? Well, your first job is to open the lines of communication. The best way to get the conversation rolling is to be open and honest about the way you feel. Get your feelings out on the table.

Perhaps you're waiting for others to approach you and offer their support. But since you're the one with endometriosis, you may have to be the first person to talk. Some people may be reluctant to even mention the word in front of you, but if you bring up the subject and talk about it matter-of-factly, you may pave the way to very effective communication.

What if you're too fearful to share your feelings? Certainly, fear can make communication difficult, if not impossible. For instance, if you're concerned that what you have to say may embarrass the other person, you may hesitate to say it. Or perhaps it's their fear that's stopping you. Fortunately, there's an excellent solution to this problem. Simply reach out and physically touch the other person. By holding hands or sharing hugs, you can quickly bring about a type of sharing that doesn't require words. In the process, you'll reestablish the lines of communication.

Jill, a 36-year-old nurse, had recently been diagnosed with endometriosis. Her family knew about it, but she hadn't told her friends yet. She decided to mention something to a few of her friends at their monthly specialty nursing association meeting. As they were discussing problem cases, she tentatively mentioned, "Oh, by the way, the doctor told me that my pain is due to endometriosis." When she saw looks of concern on her friends' faces, she immediately added, "But don't worry, I'm handling it, and will keep you posted on my treatments." The light tone of her comments reassured and relaxed her friends, and Jill felt more comfortable that they now knew about her disease.

Regardless of how well these techniques work, don't feel that you have to be too open and talk too much about endometriosis. You don't want it to get to the point where people are tired of hearing about your experiences with this disease.

Why Do Some Women Keep Endometriosis a Secret?

Some women with endometriosis may be concerned about the reactions of others. They feel that they'll be viewed differently or that people will give them more attention (or worse, avoid them). They fear being isolated. They worry about reactions from their employers. They may be apprehensive about people commenting about their difficulty in having children. They may feel as if they're becoming more distanced from friends, relatives, or acquaintances.

There are times when these things happen, but in many cases these situations can be prevented by approaching people constructively. It's best to talk to people about the issues. In the worst case scenario, you can always just let go of that relationship.

If, after all is said and done, you find that you don't have the kind of social network that you would like, it may be helpful to get involved in a support group. There you will meet people who can provide the caring and understanding you need to cope with endometriosis. (For more information on support groups, see chapter 3.)

Bring on the World

Now that we've introduced some general ideas, let's see how endometriosis can affect the different relationships that may be part of your life. Of course, not every section in this chapter will apply to you. You may choose to read only those that are appropriate or all of them. However you choose to approach this material, you'll soon realize that problems exist in all relationships, but you can cope with them successfully.

CHAPTER TWENTY

Your Family

Blood is thicker than water! Your family can be a critical factor in your successful adjustment to endometriosis. Since many of us spend more time with our families than anyone else, they can be a ready source of emotional and practical support.

Family members may experience many of the same emotional reactions you do—from anger and depression to fear of the future. Sometimes family members react more strongly and possibly even more irrationally than the woman who's suffering with endometriosis. There may be more denial by a family member. Parents may feel especially guilty if they believe that they have somehow contributed to endometriosis in their daughter. Any communication problems that exist within a family may be magnified by endometriosis.

If you find it difficult to talk to loved ones about your endometriosis, treatment issues, or your feelings, don't give up. To maintain family unity—and to make sure you get the support you need—it's important that your concerns be brought into the open. This doesn't mean that all conversations are going to be pleasant. However, they should enable each person to share his or her feelings with the other members of the family.

Of course, problems may be different for each family member. So let's discuss how you can better deal with your partner, your children, and your parents.

Living with Your Partner

Endometriosis can certainly have an effect on your relationship with your spouse or significant other. But this doesn't mean that your problems can't be resolved. Better communication, understanding, and, if necessary, counseling can help to resolve most issues. Let's discuss some of the ways endometriosis may affect a relationship, as well as various suggestions to reduce its impact.

CHANGES IN YOUR SOCIAL LIFE

Has endometriosis forced you to cut back on some of the social activities you used to enjoy with your partner, because of pain, fatigue, or other symptoms? Although this may be temporary, it can be hard to take, especially if you and your partner have enjoyed active social lives. Your partner may feel angry, frustrated, or helpless. You, on the other hand, may feel that you've become a burden.

Keep in mind that once you have your pain or other problematic symptoms under control, you'll probably be able to resume many of your usual activities. Until then, try to limit yourself to those that require minimal physical energy. Remember to take charge of your own fears, depression, and anxiety, which can also impact your relationship.

CHANGES IN FAMILY RESPONSIBILITIES

Sometimes endometriosis creates the need for temporary or permanent changes in each family member's responsibilities. For example, it may be necessary for your partner, children, or another loved one to take over some of the functions that you performed in the past. This can surely be another potential source of friction.

Eileen, a 38-eight-year-old mother of two, told her husband, Alan, that at times he would have to shop for food, prepare the meals, and clean the house—because she was in too much pain. Their two teenage children would have to help out as well. Despite the fact that Eileen's family loved her and was concerned about her health, they were understandably upset. Her husband was especially distressed since he knew little about cooking.

How can you make changes as smoothly as possible, without causing your partner unnecessary distress? First, make the changes gradually. Try to avoid overwhelming any family member. And be realistic in your expectations, keeping in mind that it takes time for *anyone* to comfortably incorporate new responsibilities into their normal routine.

How else can you help your partner adjust to greater burdens? Make sure that free time is still available for the pleasures of life. It's only when new responsibilities seem to be all-consuming that serious problems may occur. Look at any changes through the eyes of your partner. Consider how you'd feel if the situation were reversed. Think how upsetting it would be if you no longer had time for the things you enjoyed because of added responsibilities and pressures. Discuss changes reasonably and be gentle. Just as important, as these changes occur, be gentle with yourself. When you see other members of your family taking over certain responsibilities, you may feel more and more hopeless and worthless. Look at this as only a temporary situation.

IF YOUR PARTNER DENIES YOUR CONDITION

What can you do if your partner simply won't accept the fact that endometriosis is a disease? If your partner is a man, the menstrual cycle is foreign and endometriosis can be confusing, because men find it difficult to make the connection between pain or fatigue and the reproductive organs. You can, of course, try to "educate," but don't go overboard. If you're constantly badgering your partner, pointing out how things must change because of your condition, it may only cause further denial. Your partner will not accept your condition until ready to do so. In the meantime, concentrate on improving your own thoughts and feelings. Others' feelings may change, but they will do so slowly, and probably not at your urgings.

Here are some specific ways to involve your partner:

- Chose a doctor who will educate both of you about endometriosis.
- Tell your partner about changes in the way you feel in a caring, not angry, way.
- Ask your partner to read informational materials.
- Share information with another couple dealing with endometriosis.

- Offer to set up a personal consultation for your partner with your doctor (without you present) to answer questions and concerns.
- Reassure your partner that you want to feel better.
- Don't assume anything about your partner's level of understanding. Ask!

FINANCIAL PROBLEMS

Endometriosis can certainly create financial problems. Medical bills—and possibly a newly reduced income—can make things tough. Both of you may worry whether you can meet all your obligations now and in the months to come. Of course, money concerns are a source of friction in many relationships; here the problem is compounded.

What can you do? Sit down with your partner and talk over your financial situation. Try to be realistic and to reach practical solutions. Admit that new problems may arise but emphasize the fact that they can be solved as they arise. Be patient, be communicative, and above all, be positive. (For tips on dealing with financial problems, see chapter 18.)

HAS YOUR SEX LIFE BEEN AFFECTED?

As you've learned in previous chapters—and as you may already know from your own experience—endometriosis can affect sexual relations. If this is a problem for you and your partner or if you'd just like to learn more about the possible impact endometriosis can have on sex, see chapter 22. There, you'll learn how to solve some of these problems so that sex can remain an important and pleasurable part of your life.

IN SICKNESS AND IN HEALTH?

Unfortunately, some relationships have ended because of chronic medical problems. Endometriosis-related restrictions, fears, symptoms, and side effects certainly have the potential to drive a wedge into what may have previously been a good relationship, replacing feelings of closeness and intimacy with coldness and distance. Endometriosis can wash the "magic" right out of a relationship if you let it.

What should you do if your partner is frightened and "wants out"? First, be aware that certain problems may not be entirely your partner's fault. For instance, you may be too apprehensive to enjoy your relationship, and your problems may be creating a horrible package of anxiety, depression, hopelessness, and panic. If you find this is the case after viewing things objectively, get help. This package isn't one you can—or should—handle alone. Once communication breaks down, the aid of a trained professional or an objective outsider may be necessary to resolve some of the problems you have been unable to work out yourselves. If possible, include your mate in your counseling sessions. But once again, don't force the issue. If your partner doesn't seem open to outside help, get some counseling for yourself. Regardless of the results of your efforts to save your relationship, any support you can muster will only improve your emotional well-being.

IN SHORT . . .

Every relationship has its ups and downs, with problems that have to be solved. And endometriosis may make relationships even more vulnerable to crises and arguments. In fact, at some point it may seem very difficult, even impossible, to deal with your partner. But by giving added attention to your partner's feelings and needs, you will find that many—if not all—of these problems can be resolved over time. And isn't your relationship worth the added effort? Once the two of you address your concerns and make some adjustments, your partner may become your greatest ally in dealing with your disease.

Living with Your Children

Children—regardless of how old they are—need a lot of attention, help, and love from their parents. Endometriosis can surely be frustrating for everyone if you're unable to spend as much time with them as you would like. This does not mean you don't love them or you're not a good parent. You know that. Use the time you do spend with them as productively as possible, and work to help your children handle any fears or changes that may be bothering them. Here's how you can work with your children and help them cope better with your condition.

ENCOURAGE QUESTIONS

When you talk to your children, make sure you take the time to answer any questions they may have. Discussions, if handled properly, will not only be helpful for them but can also lend a special feeling of closeness.

What if your kids don't ask questions? Remember that if they really don't want to ask, they won't, no matter how much encouragement you offer. But you should tell them that they can ask you anything, because fears and anxieties can become more destructive if kept inside. Once your children know that they have the option of talking to you freely, they can decide what—if anything—they wish to discuss.

How should you answer your children's concerns? This depends on their ages and on how much detail you think they need. The best advice is to provide simple, brief answers. Don't provide long explanations unless your children ask for more information. Try to determine exactly what they want to know. This may be tricky, because your children may not know what answers they are seeking. So just start talking, and provide them with more information as they ask for it.

Should you explain endometriosis to your children? Again, this depends partly on their ages. With very young children, for example, you might simply say, "I don't feel well, so I can't play with you right now. I'd like to, but I just can't." With older children, of course, explanations can be more detailed.

Certainly, whenever you're speaking to your children about illness—especially if your kids are young—you should be careful not to frighten them. Remember that children have great imaginations and often blow things out of proportion. Foster communication by showing that you accept your endometriosis—as much as you can—and that you welcome questions.

Of course, there's one question your children might ask that will be particularly hard to answer. Whenever children know that a parent has an ongoing medical problem, they may worry and may even ask if the parent is going to die. You'll want to handle this very carefully. Children become petrified thinking about the death of a parent. So reassure them emphatically that you're not planning to die. You can say that what Mommy has makes her sick and not feel well and have pain at times, but it is not something that will make her die. This is what your kids need to hear.

If you have difficulty discussing endometriosis or your symptoms with your children, it might be a good idea to speak to a professional—your doctor, their pediatrician, a psychologist, or a social worker—who can lead the discussion.

FOCUS ON QUALITY, NOT QUANTITY

The physical restrictions brought on by endometriosis may prevent you from spending as much time as you would like with your children. To help them adjust, explain honestly to them that you may not always have the strength for certain activities. Then come to an agreement with them regarding some enjoyable things you can do together when you're feeling better. This arrangement will show your children that you're aware of their unhappiness and want to spend more time with them.

Also, try to be less concerned with *quantity*, the number of minutes and hours you spend with your kids, and more concerned with *quality*, special time during which you share feelings and pleasurable activities. If your time together is well spent, with plenty of talking and laughing, it will make up for what is missed. And as you share your thoughts with your children, you'll be helping them to handle better any restrictions that result from your endometriosis.

ADOLESCENTS

During adolescence, children begin to assert their independence. Adolescents want to start moving away from the family setting and its responsibilities. Even under normal circumstances, this creates problems in many homes. Add a mother with endometriosis to the picture, and the problem is compounded. Because of your condition, your teen may have to help out more than usual around the house. At the same time, he or she probably wants to do less around the house and be away more. How can you cope with this predicament? Well, in truth, you may not be able to change your teen. But perhaps you can learn to cope in a way that, at the very least, keeps you sane! Let's learn more about dealing with adolescents.

Don't Expect Miracles!

First, realize that dealing with adolescents is quite different from dealing with younger children—which you probably already know! Teens are far more absorbed in themselves than in their families. Remember that they are making quite a few difficult adjustments of their own and that is why they seem to have little interest in others—especially their parents! Of course, not all teens are alike. Some are less self-centered and more sensitive and compassionate than others. Certainly, you know your child better than anyone. But if you expect your usually insensitive child to rise to the occasion now and enthusiastically pitch in with household chores, be aware that you are probably setting yourself up for disappointment if you expect significant change.

Of course, this doesn't mean that you and your teen shouldn't discuss your endometriosis and any limitations you are experiencing. Talk candidly, as you would speak to an adult, as this will probably provide the best chance for a positive response. Think about the concerns your adolescent might have regarding endometriosis, and try to be reassuring. If your teen feels comfortable talking to you about your condition, encourage discussion. But remember to respect the rights of those adolescents who would rather not talk about your illness. Again, don't expect miracles, and don't be devastated if your teenager shows little interest.

When You Need Your Teen to Pitch In

Because of your condition, your adolescent may now have to shoulder more responsibilities. But will your teen be willing to help out? That's the real question!

Seventeen-year-old Ashley, whose mother had been diagnosed with endometriosis, felt guilty about not helping more at home. However, she thought that giving in would be a sign of weakness. (Heaven forbid!) This caused Ashley a lot of anguish—which, of course, she didn't want to discuss with her mom. Because of the guilt she was experiencing, Ashley escaped by spending even more time than usual out of the house—and less time supporting her mother. Ashley's mom sat down with her, and together they worked out a compromise. Ashley would not have to spend long hours assisting with chores, but she would make herself available when necessary. After reaching an agreement, both Ashley and her mom felt closer to one another—and Ashley felt a good deal better about herself.

So, you see, it may pay to take the initiative and offer a reasonable compromise. Just showing that you understand your teen's feelings may help. Perhaps things won't seem so hopeless to your child, after all.

Another tactic, too, may prove helpful. If your teen must take on some adult chores, consider offering a few adult privileges and pleasures—within reason, of course. Adolescents will usually be more willing to help out if they know that they will be treated and trusted in a more adult way.

Remember that you can go only so far in trying to get your teenager's co-operation. You can't move mountains. Continue to be as constructive as you can, putting on as little pressure as possible in order to keep the door open to good relations

Dealing with Your Parents

Parents often have difficulty coping with a child's illness—even if their "child" is an adult. If you have a healthy relationship with your parents, then you're among the lucky ones. But what if you normally have difficulty dealing with them? Having endometriosis won't help! Regardless of the nature of your relationship, consider how your parents have treated you since your diagnosis. Have they ignored or minimized your condition? Or have they smothered you? Let's look at these two possible reactions and see how you can better cope with your parents.

THE IGNORERS

Since Tina's diagnosis with endometriosis two years earlier, her parents had shown less and less concern about her condition. Whenever Tina mentioned that she had pain, her mother's response was "call the doctor." When Tina was tired, her father told her that "staying in bed won't accomplish anything." Other than making these insensitive remarks, Tina's parents had little to say on the subject of her endometriosis. They certainly never asked questions about her condition. Even worse, when she did try to discuss it, they showed no interest at all.

Parents who ignore or refuse to acknowledge your endometriosis or symptoms often do so because they can't deal with it. They can't face the fact that their child is sick. (And it doesn't matter how old you are!) Worse, many parents agonize over the possibility that your disease might have something to do with them. While this may not make any sense to you, your parents may erroneously think that they did something to contribute to your illness or that you inherited the condition. Denial might be their defense mechanism, or they may minimize your illness, hoping it will disappear.

Try to look through the eyes of your seemingly indifferent parents and you'll probably realize that this is the only way that they can cope with the situation right now. Yes, their behavior may change over time, but the change will be gradual and not necessarily in response to your urgings.

THE SMOTHERERS

After Barbara was diagnosed with endometriosis, her mother began visiting her on the average of four times a week. This would have been nice, except: (1) Her mother lived 45 minutes away by car; (2) her mother had hypertension and needed to minimize stress; (3) Barbara simply did not want to see her so often. You see, Barbara was 36, hadn't lived at home for 15 years, and often disagreed with her mother—especially regarding activities and rest. Barbara certainly felt smothered.

Parents who smother believe that if you have any kind of problem, they must take care of you. It doesn't matter what your marital status is, how old you are, or if you are extremely independent. Many parents continue to feel responsible for your welfare, and they may call frequently, asking how you're doing. They'll want to know what they can do to help. They may come over as often as possible to make sure you're okay. Whether they visit or not, they'll constantly bombard you with questions about your symptoms, your endometriosis, your general health, and probably a lot of other issues.

What can you do, short of leaving town and taking on a new identity? Again, look at yourself—and your condition—through the eyes of your parents. How do you think they feel? They care about you, and they see a child who needs them! You may not agree, but understanding their point of view should help you better communicate with them and more effectively explain how you feel.

WHAT IF TALKING DOESN'T HELP?

If you've talked to your parents and haven't succeeded in modifying their behavior, at least you know you've tried. This alone may help you feel better. In addition, you can concentrate on helping yourself feel better. If your parents are unhappy with you because you seem to be rejecting their well-meaning intentions, so be it. If they are unhappy with you because you're making it hard for them to ignore your condition, that's fine, too.

By the way, if you're unhappy with parents who are ignorers, you'd probably love them to smother you for a while. And if you don't like smothering parents, the thought of being left alone is probably very appealing. (Yes, the grass is always greener . . . !) There's rarely a perfect situation or relationship, and no one gets along with everyone all the time. So instead of complaining about your parents' faults, try to look at the positives in their behavior. This may make you feel better and will certainly help you avoid going crazy over their actions.

A Familial Conclusion

As you learn to cope with endometriosis, your biggest ally—and an important source of emotional support and practical assistance—may be your family. By learning to deal with your family members in the best possible way, you'll not only make things easier for them but also help them to help you cope.

CHAPTER TWENTY-ONE

Your Physician

Many women with endometriosis question which type of doctor should be responsible for their treatment. The consensus is that your primary physician should be a gynecologist or a reproductive endocrinologist who has specialized in endometriosis. However, other specialists—gastroenterologists, surgeons, or immunologists and healthcare professionals such as adult nurse practitioners, clinical nurse specialists, or nurse midwives, for instance—may also be involved, depending on your particular needs.

Your primary physician should be the "hub" of the wheel. She will—hopefully—be your advocate in determining which treatments are best for you, both now and in the future. She will also help coordinate the efforts of any other physicians who may be involved in your care. Your primary doctor's role is to manage your symptoms, decrease the risk of complications, provide guidelines for any lifestyle changes that may be beneficial or necessary, and even work with you when medical problems unrelated to endometriosis occur.

Finding the Right Doctor

What should you look for when choosing your primary physician—or any physician, for that matter? Clearly, you'll want someone highly qualified to treat endometriosis. Just as important, you'll want a doctor with whom you're personally comfortable. Research has suggested that the greater your comfort level, the more likely it is that you will comply with prescribed treatment and the better you may respond to treatment. And, of course, you must remember that you'll have to visit your physician more often than someone without a chronic medical problem.

Many factors will determine how comfortable you feel with your physician, including your personality, your doctor's personality, your age, your doctor's age, your doctor's philosophy regarding treatment, and more. Remember that the chemistry between a doctor and each patient is unique. Although a friend or relative may recommend the "perfect" doctor, she may not be right for you. So select a physician whom you can trust.

When screening doctors, inquire about their success in treating endometriosis. Ask, for example, how many cases of endometriosis they see every year. Request references, not only from patients but from other physicians. Keep in mind that an effective therapy for one woman with endometriosis won't necessarily be effective for you. Ask to see supportive studies, documented cases, and patients' testimonials. View all information with a healthy dose of skepticism, and pin the practitioners down as much as possible as to whether they think you can expect long-term improvement, short-term improvement, or reduced pain.

Here are a number of questions you can ask to determine if a doctor you are seeing for the first time is right for you:

- Is the doctor an expert in endometriosis, with a good deal of experience treating women with it?
- How many endometriosis patients are treated each week?
- What are the outcomes of each treatment?
- Do patients receive referrals to other specialists when necessary?
- What surgical techniques and what methods are this doctor most proficient in performing?
- What certifications does the doctor have (laser, videolaparoscopy, etc.)?
- Is the doctor's office located close enough to your home to enable you to visit easily at those times when you're in pain or have difficulty arranging transportation?

- What are the office hours? Are they convenient for you? How long does it take to schedule an appointment?
- How long will it take the doctor to call you back when you phone with a question? Will you always receive a return call from your own doctor, or will you sometimes have to talk to an associate?
- What are the anticipated fees? What are the doctor's policies regarding insurance?
- How supportive and cooperative is the doctor's staff? (You may find this question surprising, but in fact many people change doctors simply because of difficulties encountered with the office staff!)
- Does the doctor seem genuinely concerned about you as a person?
- If you have an interest in alternative treatments, what are the doctor's views on this subject?
- Is the doctor willing and able to answer your questions in language you find understandable?
- Does the doctor employ other professionals (such as a nurse practitioner or clinical nurse specialist) who will also work with you?

Of course, we all want the perfect doctor—the one with the best credentials, the most experience, the most impressive reputation, and the warmest bedside manner. (And, of course, the office should be right around the corner!) But accept the fact that you probably won't be able to find a doctor who meets all of your criteria. Determine what you feel is the most important. You may, for instance, be willing to accept a doctor with excellent qualifications but a poor bedside manner. Use your best judgment and make the decision with which you feel the most comfortable.

Creating a Good
Doctor-Patient Relationship

Once you've chosen your primary physician—and, possibly, other healthcare professionals—you'll want to develop a good relationship. Fortunately, there are two things you can do to help make—and keep—your relationship pleasant and, most important, beneficial.

SET COMMUNICATION GROUND RULES

It's vital to set ground rules regarding communication with your doctor or any healthcare professional. In the past, some physicians believed that patients with chronic illnesses wanted to know as little as possible, so they limited the amount of information they shared. Today this is not often the case. Many women with endometriosis want to be very actively involved in their treatment and to review all the facts. Regardless of how much information you want, be sure to clearly communicate your needs. Of course, this is a fairly simple matter if you want to know as little as possible or want to be told everything. But what if you want your communication to fall somewhere in between? Be aware that there's nothing wrong with saying, "Doctor, I really want all the information about my case. But please remember that I'm very sensitive, so try to tell me things as gently as possible!"

EXPLAIN YOUR ROLE IN TREATMENT

At the beginning of a new relationship with any healthcare professional, be sure to clearly explain what role you want to play in your own treatment. Some women are very actively involved in making treatment decisions. Others want to find a professional whom they can trust and then let that person take charge. Either approach is fine, depending on your preferences. Make sure that you not only communicate this but that your doctor is comfortable with the arrangement. This is vital for a good working relationship that will result in the best outcomes.

You must be comfortable discussing different treatment options with your doctor. After all, it will be up to you to decide whether a therapy fits into your own individual lifestyle, personality, and belief system. Some therapies, for instance, may require a degree of practical, emotional, or financial commitment that you are unwilling or unable to make. Some may not be feasible if you work full-time. Others may require too much travel. Some may simply be too expensive. Take time to read and gather information. Talk to others about their experiences. Then you can select a course of medical treatment or surgery from a place of strength and knowledge.

Getting the Most from Office Visits

Most communication with doctors occurs during office visits. Both parties want these visits to be as helpful and productive as possible. As you may know, this is sometimes more easily said than done. All of us have probably left a doctor's visit and realized that we forgot to ask an important question. Or perhaps we did ask the question and then promptly forgot the answer! Nothing can be more frustrating—especially since physicians are often difficult to reach by phone! Fortunately, there are ways to avoid this frustration. Let's look at some of the easy things you can do to get the most from your office visits.

MAKING A LIST

Before each appointment, it's important to prepare a list of all the questions you want to ask. Don't wait until the night before your office visit to do this. Instead, on an ongoing basis, record notes whenever a question or other detail enters your mind.

Although making a list may seem elementary, it is an excellent way to obtain the information you need to better understand your endometriosis, properly care for yourself, and guide your treatment. Don't worry that the doctor won't like the idea that you've prepared a list of questions. Most good doctors do appreciate this practice because it tends to structure the appointments more efficiently. However, if your doctor doesn't like it, ask yourself this: Whose treatment, condition, and life is on the line, anyway?

Besides those questions that occur to you, you may want to include concerns expressed by family members or close friends—even if you feel that their points may not be important. Your doctor will be able to tell you what is relevant, as well as provide you with the answers.

Many women worry that the questions they have are too simple and trivial, or even foolish. Remember that the only foolish question is the unasked one! If you need further explanation of something related to your endometriosis or a particular treatment, feel free to ask and to be as straightforward as possible. This will make it easier for your doctor to respond with appropriate information.

GETTING THE ANSWERS

As your doctor or other healthcare professional answers your questions, be sure to listen carefully. How annoying it is to realize that you've been looking at the next question rather than listening to the response! If you're worried that you won't remember everything, there are three ways to help your memory: jot down notes as each question is answered; bring a tape recorder; bring a family member or close friend.

Taking someone along is a good idea, not because you need someone to hold your hand but because two sets of ears are always better than one. Going to the physician's office can be quite stressful, so it's easy to miss what's said. In fact, studies have shown that people remember only a fraction of what their doctor tells them during office visits. Having extra listeners will increase the likelihood that you receive all important information and will also relieve some of the pressure, helping you to relax and more efficiently listen and respond. After the doctor's visit, you and the person who came along can compare notes.

If you do decide to bring a family member or friend with you, tell them what you want to accomplish during the appointment. Review the questions you want to ask and the information you hope to obtain. Your family member will then be able to intervene and ask any questions that you may overlook.

If your office visit will be to determine treatment options for endometriosis, consider having several family members attend. This will allow each one to feel involved. Of course, you and your doctor will make the final decision on how you will ultimately proceed.

Feel free to request additional information about any issues your doctor discusses. You are certainly well within your rights to question any aspect of the treatment that is prescribed or recommended, as well as any medication, diagnostic or surgical procedure, or other options. Some people, of course, prefer not to ask questions and to simply follow the dictates of their physician. This, too, is within your rights. But keep in mind that in a situation in which you want to do everything possible to help yourself, the more you know, the better.

Of course, we all want to have confidence in our doctors—to believe that they are experts in a particular field. This doesn't mean, however, that you must blindly accept everything your doctor says. For the most part, physicians respect the patient who asks questions. Don't feel you are powerless to disagree. If you are unsure of the reason behind a recommendation, question it. It's very important to be honest with your physician—as well as with yourself! If you don't like a particular treatment or if it doesn't seem to be working for you, you have the right—in fact, the obligation—to say so.

It's also important to indicate when you don't understand your doctor's answers because they're either too vague or technical. Don't hesitate to raise additional questions. Perhaps your physician only uses medical terms. Some patients may be too intimidated to ask for clarifications! Whatever the reason for the problem, don't be afraid to talk openly and honestly. And don't be embarrassed. Your goal is to talk more comfortably and intelligently about what's happening to you. If you don't understand something or if you don't agree with a treatment plan, inform your doctor.

OTHER CONSIDERATIONS

What else can you do to make your office visits as profitable as possible? Remember that you're the only one who really knows how you feel. If you think something is happening that your doctor should know about, be sure to mention it and make sure that you're heard. Don't think that any piece of information is unimportant, even if the doctor doesn't seem to be as impressed by a particular statement as you expected. Every bit of information you give can and should help your doctor determine the best treatment course for your endometriosis.

Perhaps you're hesitant about giving your doctor all the facts. You might be afraid that you'll be hospitalized if your doctor finds out how you're really feeling. You might be concerned that your physician won't like some of your "bad" habits. You might fear that you'll be labeled as a complainer who is "crying wolf" and then won't be taken seriously when an emergency occurs. You might worry that your physician will increase your medication—or not increase it! Despite these concerns, you do want your physician to provide the care that is best for you. This is possible only when you're completely open and honest about the way you've been feeling and how you've been caring for yourself.

During the visit, also make sure you have a clear understanding of any medication that has been prescribed during the visit. Be certain you know its actions, any foods to eat or avoid with the medication, and any side effects you might expect. (For more information on medication, refer to chapter 13.)

By the time you leave the doctor's office, you will, hopefully, have had your questions answered, and agreed on your treatment program. By all means, follow this program. But be sure to report any problems that may occur during treatment. And don't expect instantaneous results. It can sometimes take weeks for your body to respond to a new treatment.

Knowing When to Contact Your Doctor

One of the most important questions you'll want to ask your doctor is when to call about a problem. Which symptoms should be reported immediately? Which are not as important and can be reported at the next visit? Ideally, you should get this information as early as possible in your relationship. Ask about the specific symptoms, events, side effects, or other problems you should report, and ask the best time to call. But when in doubt, check it out. Don't sit by your phone wondering if you should pick it up; just do so. Remember that if you are taking a new medication, you cannot be expected to know exactly how your body will respond. The doctor has been through this many times and can tell you that it wasn't necessary to call at this time (and why!). After you've lived with a certain treatment, medication regimen, or some of the effects of endometriosis for a while, you'll have a better idea of when you should call.

Getting Second Opinions

Because you may not agree with everything your physician says and because no physician knows everything, you might want a second opinion and even a third! This is always important if you've been diagnosed with a serious medical problem or if the prescribed treatment is aggressive—for instance, if surgery has been recommended. It does not necessarily mean that you're questioning the initial diagnosis or treatment protocol; only that you're wisely exercising caution and want as much information as possible.

Many women worry that if they seek another opinion, they will hurt their physician's feelings. Are you reluctant to bring up the idea because you think you will anger the doctor? Keep your chief priority—your own well-being—in mind, and remember that your doctor is there to treat you and serve you. *You're* the one who ultimately makes the decisions. In addition, realize that many good physicians will accept—even value—your desire to get a second opinion. In fact, they may recommend it as a matter of course. A good physician recognizes that a second opinion will either confirm what she believes or will point out the need for further discussion.

WHOM SHOULD YOU CONTACT?

The physician you contact for a second opinion should certainly have as much, or more, experience than your primary doctor. How can you get an appropriate referral? You may start, of course, by asking your family physician or primary physician for a recommendation. If this doesn't work, you can then check with the Endometriosis Research Center, the Endometriosis Association, local support groups, or the chief or assistant chief of the OB/GYN department in hospitals near you. You can also call your county or state medical society, which is probably listed in your local telephone book. You might also have to ask your health insurance provider, who can provide a list of participating physicians. And, of course, you may want recommendations from people you know—especially from women who have themselves been treated for endometriosis.

THE SECOND OPINION . . . AND BEYOND

When you seek a second opinion, make sure that you carefully select and prioritize your questions. Keep in mind that you may not have to ask the same basic questions you asked your primary physician when first exploring endometriosis treatment options. Remember why you're going for the second opinion and focus on what you hope to learn. Then let the conversation, as well as your written list of questions, guide the way.

If the second opinion significantly differs from the first, you might try to bring the various professionals together to discuss diagnosis and treatment. Physicians often discuss their findings with each other by phone. If this is not possible, however, it may be in your best interest to seek a third opinion. Understandably, you may find this unappealing , both because of the pressure it places on you to find another qualified physician and because of financial considerations. Remember, though, that this is your life! So if a third opinion seems to be in order, by all means, get it.

Before we leave the subject of second and third opinions, remember that there is a difference between changing physicians and seeking another opinion. A second opinion serves to validate or question your current doctor's diagnosis or prescribed treatment. Nor are we suggesting that you continually shop around for the "ideal" doctor, as no such person exists. However, a second opinion can give you the information—and peace of mind—you need to select the best way to treat your endometriosis.

You're Not Locked In

Some women have a lot of trouble with the idea of changing physicians. Others seem to change physicians more often than they change their clothes! Don't use a physician if you feel intimidated about asking questions or calling when there is a problem. It's best to find another doctor if you lack confidence in the information you're being given or in the course of treatment that's being prescribed. You should get the feeling that your physiciam cares about you and has you best interests at heart.

However, before you begin looking for another doctor, carefully examine the reasons you want to switch. Are you changing because you don't get the appropriate information at the appropriate time? Are you changing because your doctor seems to lack compassion? As much as possible, try to pinpoint the cause of the problem.

After determining what it is that you don't like about your doctor, attempt to decide if your concern is valid. Be aware that just about all women who are living with the discomfort of endometriosis will experience anxiety—anxiety that can spill over into the doctor–patient relationship. Add to this the fact that physicians may not always have the answers—be able to prescribe treatments that alleviate symptoms or side effects, or accurately predict the results of a given treatment. Thus tensions may rise even higher. Is this type of tension affecting your judgment of your doctor? Or is there, in fact, a real problem that must be solved?

If the problem is, in fact, valid, you have three options. The first is to continue seeing your doctor under the present (less than desirable) conditions. The second is to be more assertive and to discuss the situation in the hopes of improving your relationship. The third option is to simply change doctors without trying to salvage the relationship.

Obviously, the first option is not a good one. Staying with a doctor who makes you unhappy is not going to contribute to your well-being.

The second option, however, may be worth considering. Many women find that talking to their doctor about their concerns in a constructive, positive way can solve problems. In some cases, it isn't necessary to change doctors. How might you approach your doctor about problems with your relationship? Don't try to do it by phone or at the end of a regular examination. Instead, schedule a separate consultation so that you will have the time to discuss your concerns. Once your doctor is aware of the problem, you may be able to reach a mutually satisfactory solution.

Perhaps you don't feel comfortable approaching your doctor this way. If you are afraid of being honest—or feel your doctor simply can't provide the care you need—this relationship may not be the one for you. If so, the third option may be the best choice.

When You're Seeing Several Doctors

It is very likely that during your treatment for endometriosis you will be working with a team of healthcare professionals. It can be frustrating if no one professional knows all the relevant information about your case. Inevitably, there are communication gaps. Even though some of your physicians may work together and try to keep one another informed, there is always something lost in each communication.

Is this a hopeless situation? Absolutely not! When communication gaps exist, either you or your primary physician can become the intermediary—the one who makes sure that each professional involved has all the necessary information.

First, whenever you visit a physician for the first time, contact your other doctors and request that copies of your records be forwarded to the new physician. Then take your own personal anecdotal records, dating back to the time you began dealing with your condition. What should you have in your records? Include all relevant information about your symptoms. List every doctor you have seen—along with specialty, address, and telephone number—and any diagnoses that have been made and treatments prescribed.

Itemize all the diagnostic tests you've received, their dates, and the results. Detail all prescribed treatments and describe the results, including both the benefits and the side effects. Record any medications prescribed, including the name, dosage, the length of time you took them, and any side effects you experienced. Any other details you feel are important may, of course, also be included.

Keep on updating this information, using a word processor, if possible, so that whenever you see a new doctor, you can quickly produce an easy-to-read copy. As time goes by, this information may prove invaluable!

In Conclusion

Your goal in life may not have been to become an expert on endometriosis. Nor is it likely that your goal was to keep ongoing records of your medical history or to sharpen your communication skills. But you'll find that your efforts in all of these areas will pay big dividends when dealing with doctors—the biggest dividends being greater health, better management of symptoms, and better coping skills.

CHAPTER TWENTY-TWO

Sex and Endometriosis

This chapter is not rated *R* for Restricted. Rather, it is rated *E* for Essential. If you are sexually active, you certainly don't want endometriosis to prevent you from having an enjoyable sex life.

The effect that endometriosis has on sex is probably one of the greatest difficulties faced by women who have the disease, and it can be a difficult subject to broach. At first, many women believe—inappropriately—that endometriosis makes them less womanly. They no longer feel like sexual human beings. This attitude definitely requires attention—and modification!

Has endometriosis decreased your sexual desire? Certainly, many women with endometriosis lose interest in sex. As a matter of fact, decreased sexual desire is quite common with a number of chronic medical problems. Is this change likely to be permanent? The answer depends on many factors. What kind of sexual relationship did you have before endometriosis became symptomatic? If you had a good one, you may have an easier time getting over any obstacles that the disease throws into your path. If your sexual relationship wasn't good, it is unlikely that having endometriosis will make it better! You may need some professional help to keep things from breaking down altogether. And if pain, medication, or surgery have created problems, some adjustments may be necessary. But hope is not lost. If you unite with your partner to work things out together, reassure each other, relearn how to please each other, and show a desire for each other, in all likelihood, you will eventually resume or continue to enjoy pleasurable sex.

Sexual problems related to endometriosis can be physical or psychological in origin, or they may be a combination of the two. Let's look at both causes and explore some coping strategies.

Physical Problems

The physical limitations imposed by endometriosis, as well as various treatments, can affect your desire for sex, your responses, and the pleasure you experience. Endometriosis-related pain or other symptoms can hamper feelings of sexuality. So can bleeding after intercourse, which is not uncommon for women with endometriosis because the thrust of the penis or artificial device can bruise or damage the endometrial growths. Fatigue, too, can be a factor. Any of these problems can result in you being less interested in sex.

Many medications prescribed for endometriosis result in "chemical menopause." Side effects of these drugs, such as decreased sex drive, headaches, hot flashes, weight gain, bloating and fluid retention, abnormal facial and body hair growth, emotional instability, depression, nervousness, fatigue, muscle cramps, and vaginal dryness, can definitely affect sexual desire and performance.

THE INTERFERENCE OF PAIN

About two-thirds of women with endometriosis report pain during or after sex. This pain can reduce both your desire and your ability to participate in sex. The pain you experience during sex may be based on where, anatomically, the endometrial lesions are located and the extent of their growth. Earlier, in chapter 12, we discussed the many ways that endometriosis can cause pain. The most common area for endometriosis to occur is behind the uterus in the area known as the cul-de-sac or pouch-of-Douglas. If endometrial lesions push the uterus into a tilted-back position (called retroversion), deep vaginal penetration during the sexual act, which can move the uterus around or pull it out of its normal position, can be extremely painful. The pain may be worse if you have intercourse during your menstrual period when endometrial implants are swollen and bleeding.

If you resist lovemaking or rarely initiate sex, your partner may interpret your concern about your illness as rejection. Obviously, if pain interferes with any of your sexual activities, it also affects your partner, who may be apprehensive about causing you pain, and this may affect spontaneity. If your partner helps you to deal with the fear of pain, you will both win.

WHAT YOU CAN DO

If your interest in sex has been affected by physical problems, you may, unfortunately have to put certain sexual activities on hold. Actually, that may be an excellent idea. Simply holding each other can be a wonderful expression of intimacy. So explore other ways to pleasure your partner and yourself. The 20-second kiss can revive the feelings that brought you together. A long, slow, deliberate kiss—which need not progress to further sexual activity—can be a great reviver of closeness. The 60-second hug helps you reconnect after a stressful day or when you are in pain. About halfway through a long hug, you will relax in each other's arms and feel a great release of tension. If returning to or increasing sexual activity seems uncomfortable or frightening, approach things slowly in order to get yourself back into a more normal routine. And be patient. Don't feel that you have to accomplish everything at once. By minimizing the pressure you place on yourself, you can maximize enjoyment and get back into the swing of things at your own pace. Feel free to experiment with various techniques and activities to determine the degree of arousal that is safe and comfortable.

Find other positions that make intercourse less painful or use other techniques to achieve orgasm. Look at a book with various illustrations and experiment with something new! For example, in the "bridge maneuver" position, the man and woman lie side by side. Both partners should be lubricated and ready for intercourse. If necessary, use a lubricant that is especially made to ease discomfort. In a heterosexual relationship, after both partners are lubricated, the man enters the woman or the woman guides the man's penis into the vagina. The secret is to use just enough depth, motion, and rhythm to maintain an erection. Additional sexual stimulation can add to the pleasure. This position provides mutual satisfaction without the deep penetration that causes pain. With any sexual partner, or even alone, any position that allows the woman to control the depth of penetration is good if you have endometriosis because you will know just when it hurts and can adjust accordingly. And before penetration, agree on a clear signal that you both know is a sign to stop if something causes pain. To help control the depth the penis penetrates, the woman can simply put her hands on either side around the outside opening of the vagina.

You can also plan your sexual activities for when you feel most comfortable. Time things to coincide with maximum effectiveness of pain medications. Allow your muscles to warm up so that they are fully relaxed. Mild exercise, a massage, yoga, and deep breathing all reduce stress, counteract stiff muscles, and enhance lovemaking. Take a bath or shower together and listen to romantic music. Always have a sexual lubricant available to reduce friction and ease painful intercourse or penetration. There are several safe and effective lubricants on the market, such as massage oils, vitamin E oil, apricot kernel oil, sesame oil, coconut oil, cocoa butter, and wheat germ oil. Some experts suggest using only water-based lubricants, because they will flush out of the system faster, reducing the risk of vaginal infection. Examples of these are Astroglide, K-Y Jelly, Senselle, and Today. If surface lubricants do not help, you may want to try products designed to moisturize vaginal tissue.

What if your interest in sex fails to increase after a period of time? Speak to your doctor, who may be able to make valuable suggestions. However, if this doesn't seem to be the solution to your problem, don't hesitate to seek help from a mental health professional or a sex therapist.

If pain or other symptoms are a problem, discuss this with your partner. Remember, men rarely experience pain with intercourse. This makes it hard for a man to understand how pain and fear of it can interfere with a woman's sex drive. So don't suffer in silence but discuss it together; you may be able to come up with a solution. You can also use relaxation techniques to help enhance the pleasures of sexual activities and decrease the pain (see chapter 12).

After surgery, satisfying intimacy can hasten the healing process. Many women find they are more comfortable with a gradual resumption of lovemaking—touching, handholding, and caressing at first as a way to express closeness until they feel ready to resume other sexual activities.

Finally, a satisfying sexual relationship can actually help relieve pain. Not only is it distracting, but sexual stimulation actually releases endorphins (chemical neurotransmitters in the brain that block pain and produce pleasure).

Psychological Problems

What's your most important sexual organ? Think about this for a while. The correct response is—your brain! If a sexual problem has no physical basis, then its cause must be psychological. In fact, the psychological variables that affect sexual activity are just as real as the physical factors. Anxiety, depression, and fear can all form emotional blocks that severely impair sexual enjoyment.

POOR SELF-IMAGE

Living with endometriosis can affect any woman's self-esteem. Do you feel like a different person? Do you feel as if you're "a damaged woman"? Are you uncomfortable thinking about your partner looking at your body? If your answer to any of these questions is "yes," your self-esteem has suffered as a result of this disease. Body image, an important component of self-esteem, plays a major role in one's sexuality. If you have a positive opinion of yourself, then your ability to respond to sex is positive. You are less likely to worry that your partner will reject or disapprove of your body. As a result, you may feel less need to limit your sexual activity simply to minimize this chance of rejection.

The development of your body image begins early and continues throughout life. During the adolescent years, body awareness becomes critical. So if you are a young woman who has endometriosis, it may certainly affect your feelings of self-worth. These negative feelings can continue as you grow older. In addition, surgery, hysterectomy, pain, or infertility might all affect your body image and self-esteem.

FEAR OF PREGNANCY

Research has shown that women sometimes withdraw from sexual activities because they fear pregnancy. This can even be a subconscious fear—one you're not consciously aware of. Whether your reasoning is conscious or unconscious, eliminating intercourse may seem like the best way to avoid getting pregnant.

Why might you fear pregnancy? There are a number of reasons. You may be concerned that you will be less effective as a mother because of endometriosis and are afraid that you just won't be able to handle the responsibility. You may be concerned that your child will develop endometriosis, and you don't want to deal with any guilt. Any or all of these fears can have an impact on your feelings about sex. (More information about pregnancy and endometriosis in the next chapter.)

OTHER EMOTIONAL INTERFERENCE

Sexual activity—and sexual desire—may be impaired by a number of emotions. It is not unusual for women with endometriosis to have feelings of anxiety, fear, frustration, anger, resentment, hopelessness, depression, loneliness, guilt, isolation, and despair. Depression may keep you from having any interest in sex. After hysterectomy, some women may mourn the loss of the removed body parts or what they symbolized. Anxiety concerning sex itself or the intimacy of your relationship can also hold you back. A woman may be concerned about possible rejection by her present or future sex partners. Or she may fear that sexual arousal will increase pain.

However, there is absolutely *no* basis for this fear! Sexual arousal itself does not cause pain, but certain positions and the act of intercourse can be very painful for many women who have endometriosis.

WHAT YOU CAN DO

When psychological problems affect sexual desire or performance, you'll want to get to the root of the cause and use coping strategies to eliminate the troubling emotions. For instance, let's say you know that endometriosis has made you feel like less of a woman sexually—a common reaction—and that this is causing problems. You have now targeted an important area on which to work. Try to remember that nobody is perfect. Everybody has flaws. (Yes, right now your "flaws" may seem more serious than those of your partner. But try putting it in perspective.) Then work on increasing your feelings of self-esteem. Focus on all of your good qualities. Concentrate on the overall enjoyment you can derive from intimacy.

If anxiety or depression is affecting your sexual well-being, you'll want to improve your attitude and attack the feelings head-on. Use some of the thought-changing procedures described earlier in the book. They may be the key to your future happiness!

If you feel that fear of pregnancy is a problem, speak to your doctor about an appropriate form of birth control. This will help you feel safer, allowing you to relax and enjoy your relationship.

What else can you do to eliminate psychological obstacles to a fulfilling sex life? A very important part of sexual relationships is communication. If you and your partner can share thoughts and feelings, you'll be in much better shape to work out any problems that may occur as a result of your disease or any symptoms or medication side effects you may experience.

What might you talk about with your partner? Acknowledge and discuss any sexual fears or problems, such as pain with certain positions. If necessary, work to alter the ways in which the two of you express your sexual desires. Fully communicate your needs. For instance, if there are times when you're in too much pain or just too tired for sexual activity, feel free to tell your partner how you feel. Talk about what feels good and what hurts during sex.

Endometriosis does not mean the end of sexual activity. Sometimes, though, it may require different ways of giving and receiving pleasure. When you can't have vaginal penetration, offer your partner an alternative sexual activity that you both enjoy. As we mentioned before, if you are in a heterosexual relationship and there are times when you cannot tolerate intercourse because of your illness, it is always possible to lie together and hold each other and let feelings flow in a warm and close embrace. The most important thing is to try new ways of showing your partner love and affection. Even when you can't enjoy intercourse or some other sexual activity, you can still give and receive pleasure with your partner. And remember that problems get worse only when you chronically avoid the issues—not when you openly discuss them and work together to find solutions.

Besides communicating your feelings and fears to your partner, you might also want to discuss any problems with your physician or other healthcare professionals. For instance, if you're concerned that sexual activity will worsen your symptoms, ask your doctor for advice on how to proceed. A qualified sex therapist who understands endometriosis might also be helpful for some couples. You can also take your partner with you to the doctor and talk about the problem openly and honestly.

Everything that's been said in this section assumes that your sexual interest or performance has been affected by physical or psychological problems and that your partner is suffering as a result. But what if the opposite is true? What if you still have normal sexual desires and abilities but your partner is the one who's afraid or thinks sexual activity may create additional problems? Perhaps your partner sees you as being fragile simply because you have endometriosis and is reluctant to initiate or respond to sexual overtures. Discuss this together. Make sure that you communicate with each other and then establish ground rules so that you know which sexual activities are okay and which, if any, aren't. And if these one-on-one attempts at solving problems aren't successful, don't hesitate to get some professional assistance. The results will be well worth the effort.

What if You're Single?

If you are single and dating, your concerns may be different from those of a woman who is married or in a long-term relationship. For example, you may wonder when the best time is to tell the person you're dating about endometriosis or your symptoms. Should you mention it right from the start, or not until you're approaching a sexual encounter? In general, most experts believe that you need not say anything at the very beginning. After all, you want to get to know the person first, and you want the person to get to know you. Then, if the relationship seems to be proceeding in the right direction, you may want to consider a comfortable time to mention your condition. If you think that there is a future with someone you are dating, you definitely need to be honest and open. It is only fair to inform that person about endometriosis. Your disease does not define who you are, but it is an important part of you that your partner will have to accept.

There are as many different ways of saying something as there are people. The one most common piece of advice, though, is to show that you're successfully handling your endometriosis. Make it sound as if you're in control. The most frightening thing for a prospective partner is the impression that you're so overwhelmed by your disease that it's definitely going to have an impact on the relationship. Test the waters first. You could say "I have a condition that involves my reproductive organs" and then watch and see how much the person can handle. Keep in mind that this is a very difficult subject for most men to deal with because the menstrual cycle is so foreign to them. If your pain prevents you from going out on a date, you do need to let that person know that you have a medical condition.

And Now, the Climax

When dealing with any sexual problems resulting from your endometriosis, remember that there are many ways to improve both your feelings regarding sex and your enjoyment of various sexual activities. As a matter of fact, in many cases, women with endometriosis feel that expressing love and passion can be the most pleasurable experience they share with their partner while going through the ordeal of living with the disease. Psychological coping strategies can help you overcome many obstacles related to interest in sex and performance of sexual activities. But the most important intervention is open communication with your partner. Even if your sex life becomes less active, you can still have a warm relationship—but not if there are bitter feelings and misgivings. Honest discussions, marked by understanding, are a vital part of coping with sexual problems, just as they are a necessary part of coping with any other aspect of endometriosis.

Remember, you must do and be what is true for you, not to please someone else. A woman who learns how to experience and direct her sexual energy for her greatest possible pleasure will improve her sex life. Have a good attitude about being sexual. If you have a loving and sensual relationship with yourself, you will have one with your partner.

CHAPTER TWENTY-THREE

Pregnancy and
Infertility

Concerns about pregnancy and endometriosis are understandable. Endometriosis can prevent conception and may cause complications during pregnancy. Many women worry that the disease will worsen after pregnancy. They may also fear that their daughters will develop endometriosis or some other health problems (such as allergies, diabetes, yeast infections, or immune disorders) often found in families of women with endometriosis.

Despite the fact that many doctors mistakenly tell women that getting pregnant will cure endometriosis, experts have concluded that pregnancy offers no protection from the disease. During pregnancy, your monthly menstrual cycle stops. For at least nine months (longer if you breastfeed) there is no fluctuation of hormones, which, remember, is what causes the endometrial lesions to swell, bleed, and scar. As a result, a woman with endometriosis who conceives may experience a completely normal pregnancy and even note relief from many symptoms. On the other hand, pregnancy may exacerbate some symptoms, such as fatigue, bowel problems, and yeast infections.

The true rates of pregnancy complications among women with endometriosis are still unknown. However, studies have reported a higher risk of both miscarriage and ectopic (tubal) pregnancy. It has also been reported that women with endometriosis may experience pregnancy complications, such as:

- Fetal malposition (the baby's face is toward the mother's front or the baby is in the breech position, with buttocks down or feet first).
- Fetal distress (an abnormal heartbeat indicating the baby may be in trouble).
- Preterm labor (labor that begins in or before the 37th week of pregnancy).
- Premature rupture of membranes (the bag of amniotic fluid in which the baby floats throughout pregnancy breaks earlier than it should).
- Preeclampsia (a syndrome of excessive fluid retention, high blood pressure, and protein in the urine, characterized by puffiness in the face and hands, persistent vomiting, severe persistent headache, disturbances in vision, or very rapid weight gain).
- False labor (light, irregular contractions of the uterus throughout pregnancy, often mistaken for true labor).
- Placental problems (premature separation of the placenta or mislocation of the placenta near the cervix instead of higher on the uterine wall).

There is some good news. In a study of 334 pregnant women with endometriosis, the incidence of premature births was low (0.01 percent). Keep in mind that every woman's body will respond differently to pregnancy because a multitude of factors other than hormonal fluctuations play a role in endometriosis.

Of course, a safe, healthy pregnancy is the main goal. For all women, early prenatal care is critical for pregnancy and delivery free of complications. This is especially true if you have endometriosis. Although your disease may pose risks, today's diagnostic tools, such as ultrasound and blood tests, can help detect problems early in the pregnancy and minimize complications.

Let's consider some of the important issues related to conception and pregnancy if you have endometriosis.

Before Trying to Conceive

You should discuss your desire to conceive with your gynecologist or other physician. This is especially important if the stage of your endometriosis is moderate or severe. Your doctor can best advise you whether this is the right time to consider conception. If it has been determined that you may have difficulty getting pregnant, it is wise to confer with a fertility specialist as soon as possible.

IF THE TIME IS NOT RIGHT . . .

If pregnancy is not advised, or, for whatever reason, you do not wish to become pregnant, the only way to make sure that you don't conceive is to use an effective form of birth control. Contraceptives available to women with endometriosis are the same as for other women. They include birth control pills (which may be part of your endometriosis treatment as well), implants, injections, intrauterine devices, and barrier methods (such as the diaphragm plus spermicide or condom). Correct use of any of these options reduces the risk of an unplanned pregnancy. It is important to discuss your birth control methods with your physician to make sure that they are appropriate and that no modification in your endometriosis management program is necessary. A barrier method of birth control must be used if you are taking certain medications often prescribed for endometriosis. (See chapter 13).

GENETIC CONCERNS

Are you worried about the possible genetic factor associated with endometriosis or that you may pass it on to your daughter? This is a valid concern.

Women with endometriosis often come from families where others—primarily mothers and sisters—have the disease. They, in turn, are much more likely to have daughters who develop endometriosis or other diseases. As we discussed in chapter 1, researchers believe it is likely that there is a genetic predisposition to the onset of endometriosis and that environment and health habits may trigger its emergence. We need more research to investigate the role of genetics and chromosome defects in the development of this disease. Until then, it is difficult to specify the statistical chances of genetic transmission; we only know that the risk does increase within families.

GETTING READY

Any woman should be in good health prior to pregnancy, but it is especially important for a woman with endometriosis. Because the disease can interfere with successful conception, it is important to learn as much as you can about possible problems, healthcare professionals who can best help you overcome them, and the options offering the greatest chance for pregnancy. If you have an advanced stage of endometriosis, and a fertility specialist has you start with an approach not usually successful with severe disease, you will be wasting valuable time and money. The stage of your endometriosis should determine what techniques a fertility specialist will recommend.

It is important for your physician to examine your entire medical history, because it plays an important role in your fertility picture. For example, if you took birth control pills for a number of years, you may not have suffered pain or other symptoms of endometriosis. Perhaps you were first diagnosed with endometriosis when you stopped taking birth control pills and found that you had difficulty conceiving. Or, if you switched to another contraceptive, you may have started experiencing pain or other symptoms and only then were diagnosed. In that case, it would be important to investigate obstacles to conception if you were interested in conceiving at a later date.

Trying to Conceive

Will you have more difficulty conceiving because of endometriosis? Changes in normal anatomy, such as scarring, adhesions, a tilted uterus, or twisted ovaries and tubes that occur with this disease can all cause infertility. In fact, 30–40% of women with endometriosis are infertile. This is two to three times the rate in the general population. If you have endometriosis, the monthly chance of getting pregnant decreases by 12–36%. However, for women with minimal disease and normal anatomy, the long-term cumulative pregnancy rates are normal.

CAUSES OF INFERTILITY

There are many causes of infertility. A woman with endometriosis may have any one or more of them. Some physicians believe that women who have minimal or mild endometriosis may have a combination of several physical and biochemical problems that contribute to infertility. Moderate to severe endometriosis causes scarring and distortion of the pelvic anatomy, which makes it much more difficult to conceive and maintain a pregnancy. For these women, if the thick adhesions and overgrowth of tissue have bound the organs in place and if the ovary and tubes are twisted out of position, normal passage of an egg is virtually impossible. The tubes can become damaged or blocked and the ovaries may contain cysts or stick to the uterus, bowel, or pelvic side wall. Any of these anatomic distortions can cause infertility.

Hormonal Imbalances

The most common cause of infertility is hormonal imbalance that leads to problems with ovulation. Women with endometriosis also typically have a shorter second half of their hormonal cycle than women without this disease. Remember, when we discussed the normal menstrual cycle, we said that many hormones are involved. The excess amount of prostaglandins that women with endometriosis produce can cause too much contraction in the uterine tubes, bringing the egg down to the uterus too quickly. This egg may be too immature to implant in the uterus. Prostaglandins may also interfere with the ability of the ovaries to release an egg. In some situations the egg develops normally on the surface of the ovary but is not released from the tiny sac or "follicle." This condition is called *luteinized unruptured follicle syndrome*, or LUF.

Insufficient Progesterone

Women with endometriosis often don't produce enough progesterone after ovulation. Sufficient levels of estrogens and progesterone help promote a fertilized egg to implant in the endometrium. If these hormones are not secreted or the hormones that cause their secretion are not released in sufficient amounts, pregnancy will not occur. These hormones are also essential for an embryo to grow.

Anatomical Defects

Anatomical defects, very common in women with endometriosis, can also cause infertility. A weak cervix is one example. The cervix is a valve that closes during pregnancy to protect the embryo. A weak cervix cannot stay closed because it cannot withstand the pressure of the embryo. A woman can be born with a weak cervix, suffer trauma, or have too many abortions, D and Cs, or endometrial biopsies that can cause this condition. Another type of defect occurs if the uterus is tipped backward and fixed in place by adhesions—a common problem caused by endometriosis. In this case, it will be more difficult for the sperm to make a direct journey upward. Finally, you may be prone to developing cysts (fluid-filled sacs) in the ovary. If this happens, eggs are not released and therefore cannot be fertilized.

Peritoneal Fluid and Cytokines

Women with endometriosis have an increased volume of peritoneal fluid, which contains a high percentage of macrophages (white blood cells that fight invaders). They kill sperm cells, which can be another cause of infertility. Macrophages also secrete a hormone called interleukin-1, which increases the body's production of collagen, a protein that creates scar tissue in the abdomen. Scar tissue can cause the anatomical defects we just discussed. Women with endometriosis also have a higher number of cytokines (white blood cell chemical messengers). These may adversely affect how the sperm and the oocyte (the cell from which an egg arises) interact as well as sperm mobility and survival.

Reproductive Tract Damage

Endometriosis can damage the upper reproductive tract. This results in many mechanical problems that contribute to infertility. The endometrial cells that grow outside the uterus and move backward into the fallopian tubes, ovaries, and abdominal cavity cause strips of scar tissue that damage the delicate structures inside the uterus, obscure the ovaries, and may cover up the ends of the oviducts (the tubes of the uterus through which an egg passes). Any of these can prevent the egg from entering the fallopian tubes, eliminating any chance of fertilization by a sperm. In women with severe pelvic adhesions where the ovary is encased, the egg may not be released from the ovary. Even if conception does take place, it may happen inside the tube, resulting in a life-threatening ectopic pregnancy that must be terminated.

Stress

Although infertility itself is a very stressful experience, in rare cases, high levels of stress can change hormone levels, cause irregular ovulation, and actually interfere with fertility. Some studies have shown that high stress levels may also cause fallopian tube spasm and decreased sperm production in men. So if you have been trying to conceive for some time, you may no longer feel in control of your body and your life plan. Infertility testing and treatments can be physically, emotionally, and financially stressful and can reduce a couple's intimacy level. Or pain during intercourse may be so severe that you choose to avoid having sexual relations. This, of course, definitely contributes to your ability to conceive.

TREATMENT FOR INFERTILITY

If you are considering treatment for infertility, it is appropriate to start with either a good general gynecologist or with a fertility subspecialist known as a reproductive endocrinologist. It is important to learn as much as you can about your doctor's training and experience.

If your doctor is a general gynecologist, ask at what point you will be evaluated by a reproductive endocrinologist if you do not become pregnant. In general, this should be after 6 to 12 months of treatment with your gynecologist. However, you should be referred to a specialist immediately if you are any age and:

- have one or both fallopian tubes blocked,
- have had other tubal problems a (such as a tubal pregnancy),
- have moderate or severe endometriosis,
- took medication for absence of ovulation for six months without conception (at any age), or
- have an abnormal "day 3 FSH level,"or if
- your partner has sperm concentration of less than 10 million per milliliters or motility less than 35%.

The Diagnostic Workup

Your gynecologist or a fertility specialist will take a comprehensive history to isolate the specific cause of your difficulty conceiving. Your physician will begin by asking how long you have been having unprotected sex and at what times in the month you have intercourse. Then the doctor will ask you if and when you had any sexually transmitted diseases and will want a complete evaluation of your menstrual cycle. She will also ask questions about your past that may give clues to the cause of your infertility. For example, she will want to know if there is a family history of exposure to hormones, such as diethylstil bestrol (DES); if anyone in your family has had fibroids, endometriosis, premature pregnancy loss, miscarriage, birth defects, or malformations. A fertility specialist will also want to know about your lifestyle. Finally, he will need your complete medical, gynecological, and obstetrical history and want to review fertility-related records from other doctors you've seen.

After taking a complete history, she will conduct a physical examination and perform several tests on both you and your male partner. These may include:

- An evaluation of the thyroid gland as well as the female reproductive organs
- A culture for sexually transmitted diseases, including gonorrhea and chlamydia
- A Pap smear
- A pelvic ultrasound
- Extensive blood tests, such as a complete blood count chemistry (CBC); rubella screen; thyroid-stimulating hormone (TSH); hepatitis B screen; prolactin; HIV screen; blood type and RH; and others
- An assessment of adequacy of ovulation
- A semen analysis

If a woman has regular menstruation (about every 28 days), she usually sees a fertility specialist in the middle of the cycle. She and her partner have sexual relations within eight hours of the visit and then an evaluation known as a postcoital test is performed that evaluates the cervical mucus and the number, quality and motility of the sperm. The doctor may also perform an ultrasound examination. The woman returns in the middle of the second half of the menstrual cycle for a serum progesterone level. She may also have an endometrial biopsy to evaluate the development of the lining of the uterus.

If the postcoital test and the serum progesterone level are normal, the doctor may suggest a hysterosalpingogram (also called HSG). This test assesses the anatomy of the fallopian tubes and the endometrial cavity of the uterus and is usually scheduled between days 6 and 13 of the menstrual cycle.

There are many additional tests used to determine the cause of infertility in women who have not been diagnosed with endometriosis. Laparoscopy is considered when there is an abnormality noted on the hysterosalpingogram or when either the history or physical examination suggests a problem with the reproductive organs. In some cases, a laparoscopy or other part of the infertility workup may lead to the diagnosis of endometriosis. A woman who has no pain and cannot conceive may be shocked when told that endometriosis is a possible cause of her infertility.

Individualized Treatment

Treatment for endometriosis-associated infertility should be individualized. There are no easy answers, and many factors must be considered. First is the length of time a woman has been infertile. As we discussed earlier, you should consult a physician after trying to get pregnant on your own for 12 months (or after 6 months if you are over age 35). If you are over age 37, some doctors recommend that you seek help immediately and not try very long to get pregnant on your own.

The severity of the endometriosis, its location in the pelvis, and the presence of pain or other symptoms are all important factors. Early diagnosis of endometriosis is critical in order to minimize the damage it causes to the reproductive system. After all, your prospects of conceiving and carrying a fetus to term are much better if your disease is mild or minimal.

If your goal is to conceive as soon as possible, your doctor will first try to correct any mechanical problems with surgery. For example, if you have a large cyst, complex adhesions and scar tissue, or distorted tubal-ovarian anatomy, your doctor may recommend a laparoscopy (to remove adhesions and implants) or a laparotomy (to excise larger or severe adhesions). Surgical treatment is best performed by a skilled endoscopic surgeon who can balance your desire for fertility with the need to aggressively excise abnormal tissue, restore normal anatomy, and treat pain and other symptoms.

Danazol, birth control pills, GnRH agonists, and progestogens have not been proven effective for endometriosis-related infertility when used either alone or in combination with surgery. While using these drugs alone does not improve your chances of pregnancy, they may reduce inflammatory reactions and make it easier to surgically remove lesions.

Some physicians may prescribe a course of GnRH agonists, danazol, or progestogens before laparotomy to help shrink endometrial lesions. After surgery, your doctor may also recommend that you continue taking them if all lesions have not been completely removed, for treatment of microscopic disease, or for treatment of pain unrelieved by surgery. This combination is most often used in women who are not currently attempting pregnancy but plan to do so in one to two years. Although at least one study found this improves pregnancy rates as compared to surgery alone, other studies have shown it to be of no benefit. There is no universal agreement among fertility specialists on this issue.

Alternative Approaches to Fertility

There are various alternative technologies to help women become pregnant once they have been treated for endometriosis. One possibility for mild to moderate disease is controlled ovarian hyperstimulation with intrauterine insemination. However, this approach may make endometriosis worse. How does ovarian hyperstimulation work? Follicle-stimulating hormone is given to stimulate the development of one or more mature follicles (where eggs develop). If there are multiple follicles and eggs, the chance of pregnancy is increased. The medication is injected daily for 8 to 14 days or until ultrasound examination of the ovaries shows one or more mature follicles. Once there are multiple eggs, intrauterine insemination is performed to coincide with ovulation by placing a concentrated semen specimen in the uterus using a very thin, soft catheter.

Success rates vary and depend on the woman's age, the total motile sperm count, the quality of the sperm, the stage of endometriosis, and whether there are any anatomical defects. In women with normal anatomy, meaning no scarring, adhesions, tilted uterus, twisted ovaries or tubes, as caused by moderate or severe endometriosis, a reasonable trial is three to four cycles. After a maximum of six cycles, in vitro fertilization (done outside the body in a laboratory dish) should be considered. Women with severe endometriosis often require in vitro fertilization in order to conceive. If a woman has a large ovarian cyst, surgery to remove it may be necessary before proceeding.

The process of in vitro fertilization (IVF) fertilizes a woman's eggs with a man's sperm outside the woman's body in a laboratory dish. The process is very complex. A woman is injected with medications that overstimulate the ovaries to induce formation of a follicle. As the follicle develops, it is carefully monitored with blood and ultrasound testing every one to three days. Before ovulation, the doctor uses ultrasound techniques to guide removal of the ovum (part of the genetic material needed for a new individual) from the ovary. The recovered oocytes (full-grown cells that are not completely mature) are evaluated under the microscope. The most viable ones are incubated in a culture medium before sperm are added. Then fertilization is done in vitro, or outside the body, in a laboratory dish. Nearly 50,000–100,000 sperm are added to the dish. The resulting embryos are cultured in the lab for two to three days and then transferred to the uterus to implant and develop into a fetus.

This procedure can be very costly. If you are considering it, there is certain important statistical and other information you should obtain, including:

- The IVF pregnancy rate for the entire program. You can ask for the most recent statistics and compare them with the results of other programs. (IVF outcome statistics are posted by the Centers for Disease Control and Prevention on their Website.)
- The individual pregnancy rate over the past year for all embryo transfers performed
- The pregnancy rate per retrieval and per transfer and whether they are initial pregnancy rates, ongoing pregnancy rates, or live birth rates.
- Information about how much any treatment will cost and how much your insurance will cover.
- A detailed listing of what is included in any procedure. For example, for IVF does the fee include:
  - All physician consultations?
  - All ultrasound and blood monitoring?
  - All facility fees?
  - All anesthesia-related fees?
  - Other costs, such as medications?

Like ovarian hyperstimulation, success rates for IVF procedures vary considerably. They can range from less than 5% per transfer procedure to an average of 27% live births per egg retrieval. Pregnancy rates are best if the woman is under age 40 and produces enough eggs during the ovarian stimulation.

Another type of assisted reproductive technology is gamete intrafallopian transfer (GIFT), a procedure similar to IVF. With this technique, the harvested eggs and sperm are placed directly into the fallopian tubes. Fertilization occurs within the woman's body rather than in the laboratory. Like IVF, this also requires overstimulation of the ovaries and the removal of the oocytes, but the procedure is less complicated. However, it must be performed under general anesthesia, which always poses an increased risk. Other techniques that you may want to discuss with your fertility specialist include zygote intrafallopian transfer (ZIFT); IVF with donor eggs, donor sperm, and donor embryos; and micromanipulation of eggs and embryos.

AND SO . . .

It is important to understand that infertility varies with each couple and so does the chance of conceiving. Treatment should be based on careful evaluation, a detailed history, a thorough physical examination, appropriate testing, and published guidelines for treatment of endometriosis-associated infertility. The outlook for success in the future is even greater with advanced technology.

After Conceiving

Congratulations. You've succeeded. You're pregnant! Now it is essential to remain in close contact with the physician who is monitoring your endometriosis. This way, if any problems do develop, you'll be able to "nip them in the bud."

Now you will have an obstetrician to take care of you. Some may suggest that you see one who also specializes in endometriosis.

So how can endometriosis affect your pregnancy? With an autoimmune disorder, certain chemicals in the bloodstream attack cells and tissues within the body. These "antibodies" circulate in the bloodstream and may never cause problems or they may lead to clots in the placenta, shutting off the blood supply to the developing baby, causing a miscarriage. Because women with endometriosis have an autoimmune disorder, this may happen.

During pregnancy, the corpus luteum produces the hormone progesterone, necessary to maintain the pregnancy during the first trimester. Some doctors feel that a "luteal phase defect" can cause recurrent pregnancy loss. This condition may occur when not enough progesterone is present to act on the lining of the uterus. This may also explain why women with endometriosis often suffer miscarriages.

As we mentioned earlier, the true rates of pregnancy complications in women with endometriosis are unknown. However, studies have reported a higher risk for both miscarriage and ectopic (tubal) pregnancy. A recent study also found a high incidence of dysfunctional labor (labor that exceeds certain time parameters established by researchers).

Possible Problems During Pregnancy

When you become pregnant you should see your primary doctor and your obstetrician (if not the same person) more often than you normally would if you did not have endometriosis. You must be that much more diligent in all aspects of your self-care.

Unfortunately, your pregnancy may not be without problems. We've already discussed reasons why some women with endometriosis may have a miscarriage. Among all pregnant women, miscarriage is very common. Fortunately, there is about a 90% chance that the next pregnancy following a miscarriage will be normal.

Most miscarriages occur within the first three months of pregnancy. This is early enough that many women don't even know that they are pregnant. To help monitor the pregnancy, a physician can obtain what is called a quantitative beta hCG after a women tests positive for pregnancy. This is a blood test that tells the exact level of pregnancy hormone present. If the pregnancy is developing normally, the level should nearly double every other day. If the beta hCG is not rising appropriately, it may indicate a tubal pregnancy. The doctor can also perform a transvaginal sonogram (an ultrasound test) once the beta hCG level is about 3,000. At this point, a gestational sac (where the baby develops) is visible inside the uterus in a normal pregnancy. Two weeks later (about eight weeks from the last period) a repeat sonogram will show a fetus and heartbeat.

Doctors can also determine if you have a luteal phase defect by performing two endometrial biopsies, taking a sample of tissue from the uterine lining. The biopsies are done a few months apart. Treatment is possible with either progesterone supplements or a medication called clomiphene citrate that can provide enough progesterone to allow the pregnancy to "take hold" during the first trimester. After that, the placenta makes enough of its own progesterone.

Besides more severe problems, the physical responses that disrupt any normal pregnancy can still occur, including morning sickness, nausea, and fatigue. Some women will find that their endometriosis symptoms may exacerbate during pregnancy. For example, you might feel constantly tired, even more tired than you did before you got pregnant. You might have increased vaginal secretions during the first trimester, either clear and nonirritating or white, yellow, foamy, and itchy. Many women with endometriosis have chronic yeast infections and secretions that may get worse during pregnancy. The hormone progesterone, released naturally during pregnancy, has calming and soothing effects. It also relaxes and slows the bowel. Your bowel movements might become irregular, both because of the pressure of your growing uterus and because progesterone relaxes smooth muscle. You may experience pain immediately prior to or during bowel movements, rectal bleeding, severe diarrhea, or constipation. Over 70% of women with endometriosis who are pregnant report nausea and vomiting (morning sickness). Other problems experienced by women during pregnancy include early contractions of the uterus, bleeding, cramping, and back and rectal pain.

MEDICATIONS DURING PREGNANCY

It is usually a good idea to stop most medications if you are pregnant. There are certain medications that shouldn't even be considered during pregnancy, such as immunosuppressive drugs. But this is not always possible. In all cases, don't take decisions regarding medication and pregnancy lightly. Even more important, don't take decisions into your own hands. When in doubt, confer with your healthcare professional.

What if you discover that you're pregnant while you're on drugs used to treat endometriosis? Your doctor may want you to stop the medication as soon as possible. But remember that you may experience a reaction when discontinuing their use.

Medication Contraindications

As we discussed in chapter 13, a number of different medications are prescribed for endometriosis. They include a testosterone derivative (danazol); GnRH agonists; oral contraceptives and birth control pills (a combination of estrogen and progesterone); and progestogens alone.

Danazol is considered unsafe if there is any chance that a woman is pregnant, because it can cause abnormal fetal development. If the fetus is exposed to danazol, androgenic (male) effects can occur on a female fetus. Women taking danazol should consistently use an effective barrier form of birth control to prevent pregnancy.

Before starting treatment with GnRH agonists, pregnancy must be ruled out because safe use in pregnancy has not been established clinically. Although unlikely, it is possible for a woman to become pregnant when taking GnRH agonists. Like danazol, these drugs are contraindicated in women who may become pregnant because they can harm the fetus. Because the potential effect on the fetus is unclear, women should consistently use a barrier method of contraception (such as a diaphragm or condom) during treatment.

Progestogens are contraindicated if a woman is known or suspected to be pregnant. The use of these drugs during the first four months of pregnancy is not recommended. Several reports suggest an association between intrauterine exposure to these drugs in the first trimester of pregnancy and genital abnormalities in male and female fetuses.

Breastfeeding

The choice between breastfeeding and bottle feeding is up to you. Can you breastfeed when you have endometriosis? Yes. Your own breast milk is recommended as the ideal food for your baby. However, some women with endometriosis are concerned about breastfeeding because of scientific discoveries indicating that we pass dioxins on to babies who drink breast milk. We do know that the longer you breastfeed, the less your hormones fluctuate, which is what causes the endometrial lesions to swell, bleed, and scar. As we've already mentioned, studies suggest that women who breastfeed often enjoy a significantly longer time until endometriosis symptoms return. If you are breastfeeding you may need to modify your diet. Be certain to discuss this with your doctor, lactation specialist, or dietitian.

Are You Pacified?

As you can see, there is a lot to know about conception, pregnancy, and endometriosis. You may have many questions about this important subject.

The best thing to do is to discuss your concerns with your partner and your physician or other healthcare professional. Everyone must get involved in the discussion. If your endometriosis symptoms return shortly after your period resumes, you should seek medical help immediately. If you wait too long for retreatment, you may have difficulty getting pregnant the next time. In some cases, women have reported remission of their symptoms after pregnancy. You are very fortunate if this is true!

What are the keys to a successful pregnancy? Awareness, supervision, and coping successfully with the problems you have as result of endometriosis. Take all these factors into consideration, and then—good luck!

Living with Someone with Endometriosis

CHAPTER TWENTY-FOUR

Living with Someone with Endometriosis— an Introduction

Endometriosis doesn't affect only the woman with the disease. It also affects everyone who's close to her. Those who are in the inner circle, and especially those living with a woman with endometriosis, are affected in the most significant way. They are also in the best position to help.

Illness can create troubling changes in relationships. If you live with someone who has endometriosis, you may now view her—and even yourself—differently. Maybe you see her as being more fragile. Maybe her disease has reminded you of your own vulnerability. Maybe you somehow feel guilty—either about your own feelings or because she has this disease. Maybe you were formerly quite dependent on her and you now have to shoulder more responsibility.

What does all this mean? First, you have legitimate concerns. And you feel responsible for this person's welfare. Certainly, research has shown that when a woman has endometriosis, her outlook, her self-confidence, her acceptance of her condition, and her desire for improvement are all important factors in the course of the disease. You want to do everything you can to enhance all of these factors and to provide her with all necessary practical assistance as well. But there may be times when it's very difficult for you. In fact you might even need to find help for yourself so that you can be as strong as you possibly can for that person.

This chapter will first explain what you can do to help your loved one. It

will then outline some ways that you can help yourself cope with the problems
involved in living with a woman who has endometriosis.

How You Can Help the Woman
with Endometriosis

If you are close to someone and she has endometriosis, you have an important
responsibility—with many components. But what exactly is your job, and how
can you best perform it? Read on!

MAINTAIN NORMALCY

When spending time with your loved one, try to behave much as you always
have. Try to minimize any changes in your interactions. We're not suggesting that
you should ignore, through word or deed, that she has endometriosis. As we will
discuss later on in the chapter, it's vital to be open about feelings and to honestly
discuss any problems. Just try not to dwell on your loved one's condition.

Why is it so important to maintain normalcy? Well, finding out that you
have endometriosis can be shocking enough, and worries about the way the
condition may change everyday life and the ability to have a family are also
upsetting. So by keeping life as normal as possible, you'll help to compensate
for the many changes that may take place and give her a stronger sense of security.

PREVENT ISOLATION

A woman with endometriosis usually has to face many problems, both physical and emotional in nature. These problems are even harder to handle when
she feels alone and isolated. Yet, in some cases, even with many friends a
woman can fear becoming isolated as a result of endometriosis. Why? Many
people may be uncomfortable around someone with a medical problem. As a
result, they find every excuse possible to avoid contact. Still others don't in-
tentionally avoid the person with endometriosis but make no special effort to
see her when symptoms restrict her from participating in activities.

Fortunately, in your position, you may be able to help. Do what you can to preserve the connection between your loved one and her friends and relatives. Speak to those people who seem to have vanished. See if there is anything you can do to reestablish these important relationships.

In some cases, relationships may become stronger than ever. Friends and family members may provide much-needed emotional support, as well as practical help. This is a wonderful blessing. But don't take advantage of others' generosity. Make sure that nothing happens to burn out these invaluable relationships.

BECOME A LOYAL LEARNER

You can help your loved one a great deal simply by learning as much as you can about endometriosis and its treatment. The knowledge you obtain will help you provide support and true understanding. Talk to her doctor, read support materials, research the Internet, attend a support group. Knowing the facts may help you, as well, as it may dissipate any fear of the unknown and help eliminate your confusion over symptoms or treatments.

ENCOURAGE, DON'T PESTER

Certainly, you should encourage your loved one to adhere to treatment regimens. But don't badger. If she is not heeding medical advice, there is a limit to what you can do to change her behavior.

If your loved one is not following her treatment plan or adjusting her lifestyle as recommended, should you tell her physician? That's a hard question to answer. You don't want to overstep your bounds. She may resent it. At the same time, especially if she doesn't seem to care about her own welfare, you don't want to sit back and let her create unnecessary problems.

So what should you do? Play it by ear. Voice your concerns, explaining that you're afraid of any problems becoming worse due to lack of treatment. Then listen carefully to her response before deciding whether to contact her physician or take other action.

PROVIDE SUPPORT, NOT PITY

Because of the difficulties of living with endometriosis and its treatment, you will most likely sympathize with your loved one and feel sad about what she has to endure. The sympathy you feel may help you provide beneficial support. But don't pity her, as this can be destructive.

Be aware that treatment for endometriosis—whether surgery or aggressive medications—can affect mood, causing depression, anxiety, and other emotional reactions. Try to prepare yourself, and resist any temptation to separate yourself. Your enduring support may be one of the most important factors for improving your loved one's emotional state. How, exactly, can you help? If you sense that she is wallowing in self-pity, just being there, reaching out and touching her, is one way. Sometimes, just by listening and allowing her to express feelings, you can turn negative emotions into positive ones. Don't feel that you have to quickly snap her out of her depression. A certain amount of self-pity can be a constructive self-indulgence. Problems arise only when the period of self-pity continues for too long. If this happens, do what you can to help restore her spirits, consulting a professional if necessary.

During times of depression, you will probably want to be as encouraging as possible. But avoid giving your loved one false hope or making false promises. It's not always wonderfully reassuring to hear that "everything will be fine." On occasion, this comment can cause more harm than good by making her lose faith in your honesty and candor.

There will be times when she is in so much pain or so fatigued that she can do little or nothing. If this happens, it is not appropriate for you to insist that she "get up and do something." That won't make her feel any better. Instead, assume some of her obligations and responsibilities. This may help reduce any pressure she feels and will certainly allow her to better conserve energy. In general, if she can do something—even if it takes some time—let her. If you feel that she is malingering, by all means discuss it. Try to make life as normal as possible for her.

AVOID OVERPROTECTION

As a family member or close friend, it's very important to tune into the needs of your loved one. Don't assume that you should be overprotective or underprotective simply because that's the way you would want others to act if you were ill. Be sure to find out what *she* wants, and try as much as possible to act accordingly.

Don't pressure your loved one. While you want to be supportive, remember to give her sufficient space to regain some control over her own life when time allows. If she's feeling better, don't tell her to get into bed and rest! Have faith in your special someone and trust her judgment.

What about accompanying your loved one on doctors' visits? If she asks, you may want to go for both support and to lend another set of ears. As discussed in chapter 21, it's an excellent idea to have four ears, rather than two, listening when the doctor explains endometriosis or details treatment options. However, if she wants to go alone and feels strongly about it, don't force her to take you.

What's the bottom line? Work with your loved one to set ground rules as soon as possible. Hopefully, she will initiate this. If not, you can start the discussion. Talk about your interest in being as supportive as possible and ask what you can do to help. Things will move more smoothly once you have a good idea of what to do and when to do it. Even if no clear-cut answers emerge, at least you'll share some constructive communication, which will lay the groundwork for handling future problems. Perhaps most important—and, possibly, most difficult—try to respect her decisions regarding how she wants things handled. Discussions are fine, but she must make the final decisions.

KEEP TALKING!

The most important key to the successful maintenance of family harmony is communication. Perhaps you and your partner have always communicated effectively, even before the pain and other problems with endometriosis entered your life. If so, you're one of the lucky ones. If not, it's imperative to establish the lines of communication and keep them open.

Why is good communication so important? This is the only way that you will learn how your loved one feels, both physically and emotionally. And only by knowing how she feels will you be able to help her. This doesn't mean that the conversations will always be pleasant. Talking about treatment problems, depression, fears, or pain isn't very enjoyable, especially if you don't have any solutions. But with good communication, any difficulties will be overshadowed by the feeling of closeness that results from shared experiences and concerns.

As much as you would like to talk to your loved one, there may be times when she is not willing to respond. When this happens, it's perfectly okay to reassure her that you're aware that she doesn't want to talk right now but that you'll be there for her when she needs a sympathetic ear.

Sometimes you may feel that it would be helpful to ask her how you can cope with the difficulty of the situation—with the uncertainties you feel and your own fears about her condition. There's certainly nothing wrong with pointing out that you're worried or even scared. Make sure you do it at an appropriate time, though. And if you see that she is getting upset, put the conversation on hold.

Take Care of Yourself, Too!

Although you probably learned a great deal about the experience of endometriosis from reading this book, so far we have paid little attention to the problems that endometriosis poses for the caregivers. There are moments when others have a harder time dealing with illness than the person who is ill. You may feel many of the same emotions experienced by the person with endometriosis but feel more helpless and out of control because everything is happening *around* you rather than *to* you. In addition, as a caregiver there are special problems that you will encounter. Let's take a look at some of the problems you may face and see how you can care not only for her but also for an equally important person—yourself!

GUILT

In chapter 8, we discussed how your loved one may experience guilt as a result of her endometriosis. You, too, may be troubled by this emotion. You may feel (irrationally) that you somehow contributed to the endometriosis. You might think that you should have been more insistent about her seeing a doctor when problems first occurred. You may feel guilty because, although concerned about your loved one, you resent the fact that her illness is going to interfere with the quality of your life. This can make you feel especially bad, because your anger and resentment are directed toward somebody who, at the present time, may appear to be vulnerable and unable to defend herself.

How can you cope with your feelings of guilt? Work to restructure your own thinking, just as your loved one who experiences guilt must restructure hers. Keep reminding yourself that you did not cause the endometriosis. You are not a bad person. You are doing what you can to help her. By reworking your negative thoughts, you will be able to reduce any feelings of guilt that might arise. (For more about coping with guilt, see chapter 8.)

DEPRESSION

Just as your loved one will sometimes feel depressed, anticipate that you, too, will sometimes experience depression. This may result from a number of things, including lifestyle changes. Accept that it's okay to feel this way. After all, it's certainly depressing when life's patterns have to change because of a chronic illness. However, don't allow this feeling to linger. Find a technique that will help to lift the depression.

Again, begin by restructuring your thinking. Depression is often caused by negative thoughts, so you'll want to follow the guidelines for changing them provided in part II. In addition, be sure to reserve some time each day for yourself. You need to have a time when you can do the things you enjoy. This isn't being selfish or negligent. Rather, by helping yourself, you'll be making yourself stronger and better able to support your loved one.

THE LONG VERSUS THE SHORT OF IT

When someone experiences an acute (short-term) medical problem—such as pneumonia, an infection, or a broken bone—it's relatively easy for friends and relatives to rally around, provide support and understanding, and temporarily take over responsibilities. But a condition such as endometriosis is a different matter. There will be times when your loved one may be able to do very little, and you will have to take on many more responsibilities. At other times, she will be able to complete more tasks and resume normal activities. These cyclical changes can create major problems. And the fact that there is no definite end in sight will not make your adjustment any easier.

How can you cope with problems caused by the chronic nature of endometriosis? Once again, work on your thinking. Long-range worries lead to long-term unhappiness. So instead of thinking about the future, do what you can each day to support your loved one and to make her life and your own as full and happy as possible. Have faith in your ability to rise to new challenges if and when it becomes necessary to do so.

A Final Note on Self-Care

You know that a woman with endometriosis needs care and support. But don't ignore the fact that you, too, need—and deserve—nurturing and caring attention. Don't be afraid to reach out and get it. Don't feel that, because you're not the person who is sick, you have to take a back seat. Your emotions can suffer as well. Remember that you can benefit from the same kinds of support groups as your loved one. In fact, there is a Website just for men who live with women suffering from endometriosis (see the Resource Groups section in the back of the book). And both the Endometriosis Research Center and the Endometriosis Association can provide additional information. Don't hesitate to take advantage of the many other resources available. To continue to be at your best for yourself, for your loved one, and for other family members, you need to be strong.

Although the endometriosis is not affecting your body, it is certainly affecting you in other ways. By following the suggestions in this chapter, you can help yourself become stronger, more emotionally stable, and more supportive of your loved one. After all, she's not the only one who has to cope with endometriosis!

CHAPTER TWENTY-FIVE

Children and Adolescents with Endometriosis

If your daughter is diagnosed with endometriosis, it is very likely that the physician in charge will immediately have two or three new patients: the child and her mother and/or father! This may only be the tip of the iceberg. When a child is diagnosed with a serious illness, it can have a devastating effect on her family. As a family, it is vital to work through any emotional difficulties you may experience as a result of your daughter's diagnosis. Remember, your attitude about endometriosis will affect her. It is important to teach her that severe cramps or pain are not normal. Good communication will keep the family intact and help make it easier for her to cope. Who else is involved? Friends, teachers, and other relatives may all be affected by your daughter's endometriosis.

PARENTAL CONCERNS

If your daughter is diagnosed with endometriosis, you will probably experience a whole range of emotional reactions. Watching her cope with the pain and other symptoms can be horrible. Feelings of guilt and intense anguish are not uncommon. Perhaps you worry that your child inherited the illness from you (or other ancestors in your family). You may feel guilty that you did not recognize symptoms early enough or that you didn't take proper care of your daughter. "Is there something I could have done to prevent this?" you may wonder. These are natural concerns, and most parents are emotional after the initial diagnosis, but these worries can be destructive unless they are re-solved. In this case, do not try to communicate your fears, which could cause your daughter to feel ashamed.

Don't let your guilt overwhelm you and affect you negatively. As in many diseases, hereditary factors may have led to the onset of your daughter's en-dometriosis. However, this does not mean that you should spend time feeling guilty. Work on your thinking. Try not to let your daughter see your pain or un-happiness. Imagine how she will feel seeing unhappiness in loved ones. You can be sure that she will feel guilty, making things worse.

Many parents find relief from support groups. Make sure that you take ad-vantage of these services and involve your daughter as well. Look for local support groups or contact the Endometriosis Association or Endometriosis Research Center for additional information.

To provide love and support, try to learn all the facts about her condition, the way it affects her, and what treatment is involved. In this way, you'll be able to do everything you can to be active participants in your child's care.

Any time you have problems because your daughter has endometriosis, discuss it with the treatment team. They are interested not only in helping her but in helping you to offer her a more loving and supportive environment.

WORKING WITH TEACHERS AND SCHOOL NURSES

It may be helpful for you to discuss your daughter's endometriosis with her teachers and school nurses. There are certain aspects of this disease that are important for these professionals to understand. You can provide them with informational materials such as brochures or videos. Hopefully, this will en-sure that your daughter can attend school without being concerned about an insensitive teacher or uninformed school nurse. It can also help teachers to intervene if other classmates don't understand or tease the child who has endometriosis.

How to Treat Your Child

If your daughter has endometriosis, you'll be much more careful in every as-pect of your child-raising than if she did not have this disease. Be certain she follows all of the components of her treatment program. However, remember that your child's healthcare team is there to support you and help make this a smooth process.

A CHILD WITH ENDOMETRIOSIS, NOT AN ENDOMETRIOSIS CHILD!

Emphasize the child rather than the illness. Avoid changing things just for her or acting as if she is "fragile." You don't want to make things harder for your child who just happens to have endometriosis. So don't behave any differently from the way you did before the diagnosis. Don't think you have to be stricter and discipline her if she does not follow the treatment plan. On the other hand, don't indulge her because she has endometriosis. Too much babying can be just as detrimental as not enough. Balance is important. In addition, try to maintain a calm, emotionally stable home. This is crucial to keep your family together and be supportive of your daughter.

It is harder to change others' behavior, but try to communicate to friends and relatives that you don't want them bringing gifts or showering extra attention on your child and that you want her to be treated normally, despite the condition.

ENCOURAGE COMMUNICATION

If your daughter has endometriosis, it's important to discuss the disease, her symptoms, and her emotional reactions. The more your child talks about life with endometriosis the better prepared she will be to become her own self-advocate. This helps to increase feelings of control, rather than feelings of being powerless, and also gives your daughter the courage to talk with others. Initially, and for a long period of time, your child is going to look to you for guidance on how to live life comfortably with endometriosis. Good communication is a vital component of managing her illness.

UNITE THE FAMILY

An important goal is to unite your family. The way to best achieve this is for parents to be united whenever possible. Any disagreements concerning your daughter or her health should be aired privately. It can be very damaging for any child to learn that she is the source of parental disagreement or dissension between a parent and another sibling. Family routines should continue as before. It may be a challenge, but each family member must learn to live with any restrictions that endometriosis may impose.

SIBLING RIVALRY

The brothers and sisters of the child with endometriosis who still live at home will definitely be affected. The degree to which siblings are affected varies, however, depending on how much extra attention she receives and how brothers and sisters react. Do the others feel as if they're losing time with you or anyone else in the family? They may feel that their needs have become secondary to those of their sister who has endometriosis. This can cause tension and resentment among siblings. Brothers and sisters may feel that she is blowing things out of proportion for extra attention. On the other hand, the child with endometriosis may not even want all this attention and may feel guilty about getting it at the expense of her siblings.

How Do Children Cope?

An important factor in determining how well your daughter will adjust to endometriosis and its treatment is how well she handled stress before the onset of symptoms. (Does this sound familiar? Of course. This also helps determine how adults adjust to endometriosis!) But having endometriosis is very difficult for a child, especially if any restrictions interfere with normal activities. You'll want to do everything you can to help her deal with this. Other problems that may occur in adults, such as feelings of isolation, pain, unhappiness with their bodies, and the side effects of medication, can also plague children.

So how do children react to a disease like endometriosis? Some withdraw, sleeping as much as they can or staying away from friends (and even family). Others are very open about their condition. They almost flaunt it, trying to get extra attention. Most children with endometriosis fall somewhere between these two extremes.

Children Deny, Too!

As with adults, children may try to deny some aspects of having endometriosis. They may eat improperly. Or they may "forget" to take their medication. Naturally, your daughter will occasionally need your guidance in understanding the medical limitations of her illness. Keep in mind, however, that there are times when children can do more than you think. In many cases, children are less sensitive to the negative aspects of endometriosis than adults. You may often be more concerned about her symptoms than she is. Try not to be overprotective. Even when she pushes too hard, allow her to be independent and learn what she is capable of accomplishing. In order to mature, your child must be aware of the limitations she should heed when medically necessary.

Some children can be encouraged to learn other enjoyable activities if certain ones are restricted. Soccer or other sports may be good for your daughter. The chapter on exercise applies to anyone with endometriosis, regardless of age. If her doctor approves of these activities, why not encourage them? Other nonphysical activities, such as chess or arts and crafts, can be good outlets for stress and other emotions. And, of course, doing well academically can be a great boost psychologically.

Getting Help from Professionals

Professionals can be very helpful for children with endometriosis. Of course, the professionals you consult with or without your child must be knowledgeable about this disease. After all, you don't want an uninformed professional trying to convince you or your child that her endometriosis or its symptoms are "all in her head" or recommending psychotropic medications. At a certain age, unique concerns might arise that must be addressed in an environment that provides coping strategies. These strategies can come not only from professionals but also from others with endometriosis, preferably in approximately the same age group, whose experiences will be a great teacher.

Special Adolescent Concerns

Ah, the joys of adolescence! Adolescence can be one of the most difficult periods in one's life. Behavior and mood swings are sometimes extreme as children move from dependence toward the mature independence of the approaching adult years.

The adolescent years tend to be sensitive ones, accompanied by insecurity and instability. Although teens can be resentful and rebellious, adult understanding often goes a long way to diffuse emotions and bring a family closer together.

Adolescents want to be independent and usually work hard at this. At the same time, they don't want to be too different. This is why adolescents may have great difficulty accepting endometriosis.

WHO HANDLES IT BETTER?

Many teenage girls with endometriosis eventually cope better than adults. Because they are young, they can deal well with fatigue or pain by resting or pushing themselves in spite of it. Many teenagers can maintain a fairly normal, active life despite endometriosis. But others may become withdrawn, depressed, and even contemplate suicide.

Occasionally, an adolescent may act differently with friends (and in school) than with parents or other family members. Could it be that she puts on a different "face" with family than with friends? Isn't that frequently the case, even if endometriosis isn't involved? Perhaps you will find that your teenage daughter is more willing to confide in you than in her friends, creating an opportunity for closeness and communication.

PROBLEMS WITH FRIENDS

Adolescents have a difficult enough time dealing with peer pressure. If they feel different because of endometriosis this can easily adversely affect their social relationships. Adolescents sometimes attempt to minimize their endometriosis symptoms or treatments as a way to show their peers that nothing is wrong and they are no different from anyone else. Talk with your teen and make it clear that this is not acceptable. However, it is far better to have your teen recognize this and voluntarily verbalize it than to force her to accept it.

What happens if endometriosis results in loss of friendships? This can be a problem for anyone but especially for a teenage girl. Making friends is probably one of the most important activities during the adolescent years. Any restrictions caused by endometriosis symptoms can have a lot of consequences. Your daughter may not be able to spend as much time as desired with friends. She may have to cancel plans at the last moment or be unable to do what her friends desire.

Leave it up to your daughter to decide whom she wants to tell about her condition. Adolescents may have a hard time deciding whether to tell friends about this disease and, if so, which ones to tell. There may be concern that this information will hurt friendships, new or old. Be aware of this and try to help if you can.

If your daughter seems to be having too much difficulty coping with endometriosis, professional counseling may be helpful. Sometimes an objective and supportive person can quickly help a troubled adolescent to adjust to an otherwise emotionally uncomfortable disease.

SCHOOL ISSUES

A teenager who has endometriosis should be able to participate in most normal school-related activities, with exceptions based on pain or other symptoms as they occur. Teachers and school nurses should be given information about the disease, but they should not feel any need to overprotect the student with endometriosis. Nor should they bend the rules. Not only would this do a disservice to your child but it might foster the very type of peer conflicts you want to avoid.

QUESTIONING THE FUTURE

As a teen who has endometriosis gets older, she may have many questions that trouble her, for example, "Will I be able to marry?" "Will I be able to have children?" "Will I be able to perform my job well enough to keep it?" "Will I be able to make and keep friends?" "Will I be able to finish my education?" "Will I be able to function as a normal member of society?" These questions bother almost all adolescents, and having endometriosis just makes them more worrisome. These questions should be discussed with healthcare professionals to provide as much reassurance as possible. Support groups and Internet chatrooms are also helpful, so a teen may learn how others with endometriosis handle these issues.

A Final Note

Adolescents need to learn that endometriosis may initially make them feel a little different. However, this can be positive. In fact, living with a chronic illness can make a teen more sensitive, compassionate, and goal-oriented. With your love, support, and education about endometriosis, this surely is possible.

On to the Future

Well, you've just about finished this book. We've covered a lot of information about endometriosis. Ongoing research continues, and new, more effective medications, surgical procedures, and other interventions are being discovered. These will all serve to further improve quality of life for women of all ages who suffer with endometriosis.

Perhaps by the time you read this, some drug or treatment will have proven even more successful than the ones discussed here. It remains to be seen what new developments may improve your life with endometriosis. But it's very reassuring that many experts continue to search for ways to help the millions of women who suffer.

Although it would be impossible to discuss every conceivable problem related to endometriosis, hopefully what you've read will help you develop your own strategies for coping. Because things change and what troubles you one day may not bother you the next (and vice versa), use this book as a resource: whenever you have questions or concerns, consult the appropriate section. If you have any comments, information that you feel is important, or additional questions, feel free to write to us in care of Penguin Putnam Inc., Attention: Avery, 375 Hudson Street, New York, NY 10014. We'd be happy to hear from you.

As we said at the very beginning of the book, until such time as there is no longer a medical condition called endometriosis, keep on coping the best you can. Look brightly ahead, act proudly, and enjoy life as best you can. Remember that despite endometriosis, you can *always* improve the quality of your life!

Surgery Preparation Lists

Getting Ready for Surgery

Any surgery, particularly a major procedure (such as a laparotomy or hysterectomy) can be frightening. The more you know about the surgery itself, the consequences of anesthesia, and your postoperative recovery period, the less scared you will be. After all, if you know that something you are experiencing after surgery is normal, you won't have to worry that something has gone wrong. You might also let the surgeon know your preferences regarding incision, suturing, and other important issues. A good, caring physician will openly discuss all of your concerns and let you make certain decisions whenever possible. So, for any surgical procedure, here is a list of things that you may want to discuss with both the surgeon and the anesthesiologist:

WHAT TO DISCUSS WITH THE SURGEON

- What is the reason for your surgery and what exactly will be done?
- What type of incision will be necessary (vertical, horizontal, bikini cut), and do you have a choice?

- How will the surgery be performed?
- What suturing technique (staples, sutures, internal sutures, and steristrips) will be used, and do you have a choice?
- Can something be done to help prevent adhesions (such as using surgical implants)? What are the advantages and disadvantages of this?
- Will a sequential compression device (a pump that enhances blood flow in your legs) be applied during surgery and afterward? (There is always the possibility of complications after surgery. It is important to prevent an embolism or blood clot.)
- Will you be given a course of IV antibiotics to prevent another complication of surgery—a postoperative wound infection?
- How much pain is expected after the surgery and how can it be managed? (Options often include epidural anesthesia and/or a patient-controlled pump administration of pain medication into your vein. After the first 24 to 48 hours you may do well with oral pain medication.)
- What specific techniques will the surgeon use to remove the cysts, endometriosis, adhesions, or other problems?
- Are you at high risk for any complications? If so, why, and what are they?
- How do you expect to deal with any unforeseen complications should they arise?
- What will be used to prepare your bowel? (Usually, you follow a liquid diet for two days before surgery and then take a liquid bowel stimulant and/or enema to thoroughly clean out the contents.)
- Will your surgeon do a bowel resection or other procedures if required? If not, will there be a colorectal or other surgeon assisting?
- Do you prefer to be awake and talk to the surgeon before receiving anesthesia? (Be sure that the surgeon communicates this to the anesthesia department. Otherwise you may receive medication that makes you drowsy or gives you amnesia before going into the operating room.)
- If present during surgery, what will be the role of interns or residents? (If you do not specify that you only want your surgeon doing

the complete procedure, they may perform the surgery or any portion of it.)

- If you have arthritis, an artificial joint, or need special positioning,
  be sure to tell the surgeon.
- In which hospital does the surgeon have privileges? Can you choose
  the hospital?
- How long is the normal length of stay in the hospital?
- What does the surgeon expect will be *your* length of stay?
- Do you need to store some of your blood?
- What are your postoperative restrictions?
- When can you expect to return to work and normal activities?
- When can you expect to engage in sexual intercourse?
- When can you expect to return to a normal exercise regimen?
- What pre-op tests are needed?
- When and where will the pre-op tests be done?
- Has your surgeon received approval from your insurance company
  for all procedures?
- Will you receive a prescription for painkillers before surgery so you
  can have it filled in advance?

WHAT TO DISCUSS WITH THE ANESTHESIOLOGIST OR NURSE ANESTHETIST

- Be prepared to provide your previous history and family history with
  anesthesia (include any allergies, side effects, nausea, vomiting,
  previous surgeries and family members' surgeries).
- Give a complete medical history, including all illnesses, diseases,
  and past surgeries.
- Be honest regarding your use of tobacco and alcohol.
- Name all drugs you take (prescription, over-the-counter, herbs, vitamins, minerals, supplements).
- List all allergies (drugs, food, pollen, etc.).

- What can be done to reduce the chances of postoperative nausea or vomiting?
- What is the anesthesia you will use? This starts with an inducer (to make you sleepy) and then a gas is administered. You may also have epidural anesthesia (administered through the spine).
- Reiterate that you want to be alert and not drugged when you go to the operating room (if this is your choice).
- Can you be positioned during anesthesia so arthritis or any other problems are not aggravated?
- Will there be any followup for pain management? (This should occur if you had an epidural as well as general anesthesia.)

WHAT TO DISCUSS WITH YOUR HEALTH INSURANCE REPRESENTATIVE

It's not enough that you want to get everything clarified with the doctors and healthcare professionals. Chances are you also have to deal with your insurance company. In fact, this is a good idea, so there are no surprise "denials" after your procedure. Here is a list of items for consideration:

- Have they approved all procedures and tests?
- What documentation do they require for payment?
- Can you have a private room? What would it cost? (You may find that when you go to the hospital admitting department, they will answer this question. Often it can be only a few dollars extra that you pay out-of-pocket. If you can afford it, it is certainly nice to have the privacy after major surgery.)
- What out-of-pocket expenses will you have to pay ?
- If your doctor has trouble getting surgery approved by the insurance company, you will need to document your treatment history, including past medical and surgical treatments that were less expensive or that failed.

- Will they pay for implants to reduce risk of adhesions that would require surgery at a later date?
- Is there a way to reduce cost (for example, recent lab work or x-rays may not need to be repeated in pre-op workup)?

After Surgery

Many women go into surgery unaware of the many events that normally occur after anesthesia. Each person's experience will be unique, but there are many normal side effects that should not worry you. And the nursing staff will be keeping a close watch on you. The aftereffects will be less of a problem if you have outpatient surgery (such as a laparoscopy) than if you have a major procedure (such as a laparotomy or hysterectomy). Before surgery, review the list with your doctor so that you are prepared and know what to expect. Here is a list of many possible things you might experience:

WHAT YOU MIGHT EXPECT FROM SURGERY AND ANESTHESIA

- Dry mouth or tenderness on the roof of your mouth (ask for a swab, wet cloth or ice)
- Cracked lips (ask for petroleum jelly)
- Nausea, vomiting
- Pressure and tenderness over your abdomen and pelvic area
- Dizziness or feeling "lightheaded" when you first get up
- Bloating and gas (ask for medication to help)
- Constipation
- Nurses frequently checking your blood pressure and other vital signs

- Oxygen cannula (a tube with two prongs that is inserted into your nostrils)
- IV for fluids, drugs (it will be started before the surgery)
- Tape pulling your skin where the IV is in place
- A catheter in your bladder to drain urine
- No food or water for a certain period of time
- Fluctuation in temperature (normal if not over 100.5°F)
- Shivering from the cold
- Hot flashes
- Numbness in legs with epidural anesthesia
- Thick mucus coming up from your lungs
- Black-and-blue areas around your incision
- Itching (side effect of anesthesia)
- No sleep the first night
- Urinary burning first day after catheter is removed
- Bladder spasms after catheter is removed
- Being offered (or needing) an enema, stool softener, and/or suppository for bowels
- Drainage from the vagina
- Burning in the back of your throat when you drink liquids
- Hiccups
- A good half day and a bad half day
- Dry skin, hair loss, brittle nails (for up to one year)
- Feeling like a truck ran over you

WHAT IS NOT NORMAL

Complications are rare, but sometimes things do go wrong. These events may sound frightening to you, especially if you have never been in a hospital. Yes, the experience can be stressful, but the goal is to be prepared when you enter the hospital so you will be less fearful. Remember that these events are RARE and are not necessarily life-threatening, but you should report them to your doctor or nurse.

- Pain at the IV site
- Fluid leaking from the IV site
- Fluid going into your tissues at the IV site
- Bleeding from an incision
- Green sputum
- Shaking uncontrollably
- Very high fever
- Pain not controlled by medication
- No bowel movements
- Vomiting after you are discharged

GETTING BACK ON YOUR FEET AGAIN

Finally, you can do a few simple things to make your hospital experience a little easier. Some of these suggestions are to help prevent complications and get you back on your feet as fast as possible. Others just may make you feel a little more comfortable.

- As soon as you are awake and whenever you think of it, move your toes and legs.
- Move side to side in bed to increase circulation and prevent blood clots.
- Sit on the side of the bed (ask for help if you need it) and dangle your legs.
- Do your breathing exercises to loosen secretions (the nurse will give you a little plastic device).
- Cough after taking three deep breaths.
- Get out of bed and walk (with help) to dissipate gas and get your bowels moving.
- Drink lots of liquids.
- Get pain medicine when you need it.
- Have someone give you a back rub.

- Get flowers: it helps to know people care, and they cheer up the hospital room.
- Take a walk down the hall with someone you love.
- Take a shower as soon as you receive permission.
- Use your favorite body lotion, keep your face moisturized, brush your hair.
- Listen to music (have your favorite tapes and a portable tape player to soothe and relax you).
- Cut your toenails before surgery (you won't be able to reach them for awhile afterward).
- Use mouthwash to refresh your dry mouth.
- Take deodorant and use it.
- Arrange for help for at least the first week when you go home.
- When you get home, diffuse essential oils that help calm and relax.
- Rest and sleep whenever your body tells you to.

Further Reading

The following resources, which provide more information on the material presented in this book—and focus on other topics, as well—may help you cope with various aspects of living with endometriosis. By no means should you limit yourself to those listed here. Many other publications examine endometriosis treatment, nutrition, the challenges of living with chronic illness, and other subjects that may be of interest to you. Don't hesitate to take advantage of all the information available at your local library or bookstore, from professional associations and support groups, and on the Internet.

In addition, the authors have provided endometriosis sufferers with a unique accompaniment to this in-depth resource. *Successful Living with Endometriosis* is a motivating action workbook that provides simple yet effective strategies for living well in spite of this disease. This page-by-page guide takes a positive, empowering approach to help endometriosis sufferers improve their emotional and social well-being, and includes techniques to help enhance self-esteem and improve relationships with family, friends, colleagues, and healthcare professionals. For more information or to obtain your copy of *Successful Living with Endometriosis*, please contact Balance Enterprises by phone at 516-822-3183 or email them at BALANCEENT@aol.com.

Achterberg, J., B. Dossey, and L. Kolkmeier. *Rituals of Healing: Using Imagery for Health and Wellness.* New York: Bantam Books, 1994.

Balch, J., and P. Balch. *Prescription for Nutritional Healing.* New York, NY: Avery, 2000.

Ballweg, M. L., and the Endometriosis Association. *The Endometriosis Source Book.* Chicago: Contemporary Books, 1995.

Betler, R., and M. Lewis. *Love and Sex After Forty.* New York: Harper and Row, 1986.

Burton Goldberg Group. *Alternative Medicine: The Definitive Guide.* Tiburon, CA: Future Medicine, 1999.

Fanning, P. *Visualization for Change.* Oakland, CA: New Harbinger, 1988.

Gladstar, R. *Herbal Healing for Women.* New York: Simon and Schuster, 1993.

Lazarus, A. *In the Mind's Eye.* New York: Rawson, 1977.

Lininger, S. *The Natural Pharmacy.* Rocklin, CA: Prima, 1998.

Matthews-Simonton, S., and R. Shook. *The Healing Family.* New York: Bantam Books, 1984.

Mills, D. S., and M. Vernon. *Endometriosis: A Key to Healing Through Nutrition.* Boston: Element Books, 1999.

Northrup, C. *Women's Bodies, Women's Wisdom: Creating Physical and Emotional Health and Healing.* New York, NY: Bantam Books, 1994.

Phillips, R., and G. Motta. *Successful Living with Endometriosis: An Action Workbook.* Hicksville, NY: Balana, 2000.

Worwood, V. *The Complete Book of Essential Oils and Aromatherapy.* San Rafael, CA: New World Library, 1991.

Resource Groups

The following groups can provide you with more information on endometriosis, suggest helpful books and videos, direct you to support groups, and inform you of other valuable services. Feel free to contact these organizations and take advantage of their expertise.

Endometriosis Association
International Headquarters
8585 N. 76th Place
Milwaukee, WI 53223
414-355-2200
800-992-3636
www.EndometriosisAssn.org
email:
  endo@endometriosisassn.org

Endometriosis Research Center
630 Ibis Drive
Delray Beach, FL 33444
800-239-7280
www.endocenter.org
email: ERC Webmaster

American Academy for Guided
  Imagery
P.O. Box 2070
Mill Valley, CA 94942
800-726-2070

American Association of
Acupuncture and Oriental
Medicine and
American Holistic Medical Asso-
ciation
4101 Lake Boone Trail, Suite 201
Raleigh, NC 27607
919-787-5181

American Association of Naturo-
pathic Physicians
2366 Eastlake Ave., Suite 322
Seattle, WA 98102
206-323-7610

American Chronic Pain Association
P.O. Box 850
Rocklin, CA 95677
916-632-0922

American College of Obstetri-
cians & Gynecologists
409 12th Street, S.W.
Washington, D.C. 20024
202-638-5577

American Institute of Hypnotherapy
1805 East Garry Avenue, Suite
100
Santa Ana, CA 92705
714-261-6400

American Massage Therapy Association
820 Davis Street, Suite 100
Evanston, IL 60201
312-761-2682

American Society for Reproductive Medicine
1209 Montgomery Highway
Birmingham, AL 35216
205-978-5000
www.asrm.com

American Society of Clinical
Hypnosis
2200 East Devon Avenue, Suite
291
Des Plaines, IL 60018
708-297-3317

Association for Applied Psychophysiology and Biofeedback
10200 West 44th Avenue, Suite
304
Wheat Ridge, CO 80033
303-422-8426

Association of Reproductive
Health Professionals
2401 Pennsylvania Ave., N.W.,
Suite 350
Washington, DC 20037
202-466-3825

Bio-Electro-Magnetics Institute
2490 West Moana Lane
Reno, NV 89509
702-827-9099

Candida and Dysbiosis Information Foundation
409-694-8687

American Association for Chronic
Fatigue Syndrome
c/o Harborview Medical Center
325 Ninth Ave.
Box 359780
Seattle, WA 91804
206-521-1932
www.accfs.org

HERS Foundation (Hysterectomy
Educational Resources and
Services)
4222 Bryn Mawr Ave.
Bala Cynwyd, PA 19004
215-667-7757
www.dca.net/~hers/

International Academy for
Compunding Pharmacists
P.O. Box 1365
Sugar Land, TX 77478
800-927-IACP
www.IACPRX.org

International Medical and Dental
Hypnotherapy Association
4110 Edgeland, Suite 800
Royal Oak, MI 48073
313-549-5594
800-257-5467

Interstitial Cystitis Association of
America
51 Monroe, Suite 1402
Rockville, MD 20850
800-435-7422
www.ichelp.org

National Association for Holistic
Aromatherapy
P.O. Box 17622
Boulder, CO 80308
303-258-3791

National Center for Homeopathy
801 North Fairfax, Suite 306
Alexandria, VA 22314
703-548-7790

National Chronic Pain Outreach
Association
822 Wycliffe Court
Manassas, VA 22110
703-368-8884

National Guild of Hypnotists
P.O. Box 308
Merrimack, NH 03054
603-429-9438

Office of Alternative Medicine
National Institutes of Health
OAM Clearinghouse
P.O. Box 8218
Silver Spring, MD 20907
888-644-6226

INTERNATIONAL ORGANIZATIONS

Endometriosis Association of
    Australia (Victoria)
37 Andrew Crescent
South Croydon
Victoria, Australia 3136
phone: 61 3 9870 0536

Japan Endometriosis Association
5060-2-302
Nakano, Nakano-Ku
phone: 81 3 3228 9960

National Endometriosis Society
50 Westminister Palace Gardens
Artillery Row
London SW1P 1RL England
phone: 0171 222 2781
www.endo.org.uk/

New Zealand Endometriosis
    Foundation
P.O. Box 1683
Palmerston North
phone: 06 359 2613
Ob/gyn Endometriosis Pavilion
www.obgyn.net/endo/update.htm

North West Tasmanian En-
    dometriosis Support Group
GPO Box 1954
Hobart 7001
Tasmania, Australia

ONLINE RESOURCES

Center for Disease Control Statis-
    tics on Assisted Reproductive
    Technology Success Rates
www.cdc.gov

Endometriosis Pavilion and Endo
    Zone
www.obgyn.net

To find a doctor who is an endometriosis specialist:
www.womenssurgerygroup.com

Infertility Online
www.infertilityonline.com

International Adhesions Society
www.adhesions.org

MENDO: Men and Endometriosis
Electronic Newsletter
www.oghyn.net/endo/articles/
mendo-news-0.1htm

International Pain Society
www.pervicpain.org

American Academy of Pain Management
www.aapainmanage.org

Center for Endometriosis Care
(Dr. Robert Albee)
www.centerforendo.com
www.pelvicpain.com

Dr. Cook's Endometriosis and
Pelvic Pain Information Page
www.drcook.com

St. Charles Medical Center (Dr.
Redwine)
www.empnet.com/scmc/endo/html

The Endometriosis Care Center at
Dunwoody Medical Center
www.dunwoodymed.com/endo

Dr. Camran R. Nezhat
www.nezhat.com

Society of Laparoendoscopic Surgeons
www.sls.org

The Medicine Program
www.themedicineprogram.com/
info.html

The Endometriosis Calendar
www.thriveonline.com/health/end
o/tools.Calendar.art.html

The Pain Map
www.thrivesonline.com/health/
endo/tools.worksheet.
painmap2.html

Index